~

ENDOMETRIOSIS— ONE WOMAN'S JOURNEY

Jennifer Marie Lewis

The Griffin Publishing Group
Glendale, California

~

This book is in no way intended to be a substitute for the advice of a personal physician regarding medical matters. The author and the publisher disclaim any liability or loss, personal or otherwise, resulting from the information in this book.

~

Publisher: Robert Howland
Director of Operations: Robin Howland
Managing Editor: Marjorie L. Marks
Book Design: Mark M. Dodge
Cover Design: Big Fish
Contributing Editors: Janet Eastman & Mary Lou Elders
Photos Provided by Atlanta Reproductive Health Centre

10 9 8 7 6 5 4 3 2 1

ISBN 1-882180-91-7

Griffin Publishing Group
544 Colorado Street
Glendale, California 91204

Telephone: (818) 244-1470

This book is dedicated to my mother, Carol, without whose strength and support this book could never have been written.

ACKNOWLEDGMENTS

Special appreciation is given to James Lewis, M.D. F.A.C.O.G., and Lisa Sandles, M.D., who took a chance and gave me my life back. I would also like to acknowledge the consistent support and strength of my mother, Carol Lewis, who held it all together when I was falling apart. I would like to thank my wonderful, tolerant and incredible therapist, Sande Kiriluk, M.F.C.C., for helping me find the strength within to carry on.

Thank you to the women who took the time to share their most intimate and invaluable experiences. To all women with endometriosis, you are the true heroes.

Above all, I would like to thank God for giving me strength and, in times of total chaos, doing for me what I could not do for myself.

CONTENTS

~

FOREWORD

Mark Perloe, M.D.

Jennifer Marie Lewis has given a face, a name and, most important, a sincere voice to the personal pain of endometriosis. By sharing her medical saga and the lessons she has learned, Jennifer encourages all women to become involved as active partners in making medical decisions about the care of their bodies.

Perhaps the most important lesson this book offers its readers is the knowledge that each endometriosis case is unique. No single treatment fits everyone. While many physicians have surgical skills and medical knowledge, it is impossible to make decisions about appropriate therapies without the patient as a partner. A doctor may recommend pregnancy; the patient may not be ready to become a parent. The doctor may recommend a hysterectomy; the patient may want to have children.

There is no standard treatment or surgical procedure for endometriosis. Rather, how a woman lives her life, consideration of her childbearing goals, whether she has pain with intercourse or at intervals during her monthly cycle—these and other issues must be factored into treatment recommendations.

A misunderstood and frequently misdiagnosed or underdiagnosed disorder, endometriosis occurs when endometrial fragments attach to nearby pelvic structures and grow. No one has provided a coherent theory to explain all cases. Similarly, there is no certainty about whether the immunologic changes in women with endometriosis cause the disorder or result from it.

What we do know is that endometriosis affects more than 5 million American women, 30 percent to 40 percent of whom are infertile, in very individual ways that seriously interfere with the quality of their lives. Endometriosis crosses all demographic and age boundaries, often manifesting during puberty with painful menses. More than a decade later, after years of hurting and maybe the distress of infertility, a laparoscopic procedure will confirm an endometriosis diagnosis.

Unfortunately, there are no good data on the impact of endometriosis as a public health problem, in part because of often delayed diagnosis and the nightmare of misinformation, myths and problematic hit-and-miss treatments.

However, there is good news. The National Institutes of Health have made endometriosis research a priority in the Office of Research on Women's Health and the National Institute of Child Health and Human Development. Through research funded by government grants, we'll begin to understand the public health ramifications of endometriosis and improve both diagnosis and treatment options. But this will take time.

Until we have answers from such research, the story of Jennifer Lewis' journey will encourage more women to take up the mantle of responsibility for their health care. Jennifer learned the difficult way that a woman's doctor should be her advocate, her teacher and her health care partner. A doctor should respect the patient and be concerned with her quality of life. As Jennifer says, a patient should never blindly follow the embroidered M.D. on the sterile white coat without questioning the person inside.

Jennifer challenges women to find an endometriosis medical specialist who knows the scientific literature and to build a long-term trusting relationship with that person. The physician should be willing to listen and share his or her knowledge. Whether the physician is around the corner or across the country, every woman is entitled to a doctor-patient relationship that makes her feel comfortable and provides compassionate, state-of-the-art care for a complex disease.

Endometriosis is not a one-size-fits-all diagnosis. Rather, as a disorder with still-primitive diagnosis stages, treatment must be individualized to each woman's symptoms, disease progression and personal needs. Care usually involves ongoing adjustment of treatments that may include, but are not limited to, surgery, hormones or hormone suppressants and pain control, in addition to emotional support, counseling and assertiveness training to help each patient focus on her needs and how to express them.

A diagnosed woman is entitled to information. Physicians not only should answer questions but also make sure the patient understands those answers. An effective partnership begins with knowing what questions to ask. For example, if the doctor prescribes a pain medication or hormone, the patient should ask:

~ How long will it take to work?
~ At what point will we know if the medication is not working?
~ What if the prescription doesn't work?
~ What are the side effects—short-term and long-term?
~ If the drug is effective, how long can it be safely used?
~ What are the options after the drug?
~ What if I wake up at night in terrible pain?

If surgery is recommended as part of the treatment plan, it should be performed only by a skilled endoscopic surgeon who is comfortable with all the medical options and psychological ramifications of endometriosis therapy. The physician also should be experienced in managing infertility and, equally important, be open to listening to his or her patient's concerns.

The glitter of new technology such as laser, electrosurgery or microbipolar instruments matters less than the surgeon's skill. Even surgical scissors can be effective if the surgeon works aggressively to excise all visible disease. The surgeon should also take preventive steps during surgery to minimize the risk of adhesions.

Earlier studies questioned the value of surgical treatment for minimal endometriosis. More recent data have shown increased pregnancy rates as a result of early intervention. Considering the progressive nature of this disorder, the latest research appears to confirm the value of aggressive management at the time of diagnosis as a means of controlling disease progression.

Along with medical treatment and support groups, a good pain management counselor also may be helpful. The simple truth is that endometriosis hurts. And pain can make every aspect of life difficult while undermining a woman's ability to relate to others.

A crucial element in the total care picture is to have a partner who is willing to listen and understand how endometriosis affects them as a couple, as well as each of them as individuals. An experienced counselor can encourage communication skills and assertiveness without aggressiveness.

Whatever combination of surgery, hormonal therapy, pain medication and psychological support a doctor recommends, Jennifer Lewis believes that medical care should not be done *to* a woman but, rather, *with* her. When the patient is an active partner with her physician in making treatment decisions, the goals of alleviating pain, slowing disease progression and restoring fertility, if possible, often can be met.

Mark Perloe, M.D.
Atlanta Reproductive Health Care Centre
June 9, 1997

~

INTRODUCTION

I was 15 and naive when I began experiencing severe menstrual pains and unpredictable, intermittent bleeding. With each month the severity and magnitude of my pain and spotting increased. It was summer 1984 and all I knew about my menses was what my mother had prepped me for by briefly explaining: There would be discomfort, but no real pain, accompanied by moderate bleeding about every 28 days. I was unprepared for what was happening. The only fact I was sure of was that I faced debilitating pain, frustration and fear. In search of information and a cure, I encountered many gynecologists who dismissed my pain as a stretched muscle caused by exercise or a young girl's imagination.

Could I be exaggerating disproportionately the pain that by then had kept me home and away from school, sports and parties? I could not attend most events loved by teenagers because of unmanageable bleeding and extreme pain. These episodes were embarrassing and disruptive to both my body and my self-esteem.

By the time I was 17, my mother and I had been flying from doctor to doctor with no concrete explanation for the pain. Because I had some rough years growing up (weight problems and unpopularity, which led to a great dislike of school and few friends), some doctors thought psychological trauma was causing the pain in my lower abdomen. Another dismissal, this time with a harsh name: psychosomatic. They said I had to change my mind, not my body. I was devastated. I was crying for help with none being offered.

At 18, I went to a gynecologist and explained my plight, begging for some compassion. It had been three years of misdirection, and my resolve had turned to hopelessness. I sat with the gynecologist and he taught me a new word: Endometriosis.

He explained that endometriosis occurs when bits of the endometrium (the tissue that lines the uterus) escape the uterus and become implanted on other pelvic organs, most often the ovaries, uterus, Fallopian tubes or supporting ligaments of the uterus. These mislocated cells imitate the menstrual cycle, first thickening and then bleeding.

Because the implants are embedded within otherwise normal tissue, there is no place for the blood to flow. They form blood blisters, irritating the surrounding tissue, which may create a cyst to encapsulate the blister. The cyst, in turn, may become a scar or an adhesion. This can cause extremely painful menses and disrupt a woman's regular cycle.

Endometriosis. I could barely pronounce the word, let alone believe that a doctor had finally opened a door to diagnosing my condition. I had to learn more. I had to learn if I had this. The only way to determine if a woman has endometriosis is with exploratory surgery called a laparoscopy.

A laparoscope is a slim instrument equipped with a light. It is inserted into the abdomen through a small incision, and the physician looks through it to examine areas of the abdomen where endometrial implants may lie. Once found, these implants can be cauterized, excised or burned with laser technology where physicians "zap" the implant with a laser beam instead of physically manipulating the area. Which technique is used depends on the individual. These techniques will be explained in depth later in the book.

As much as I had been searching for answers to my years of pain, I was overwhelmed. Could this be it? I had so many questions, so many fears. Did I have cancer? Could I have children? Would I have to be cut open? And, most of all, would this cure me?

I began to imagine a light at the end of the tunnel. The light was quickly dimmed when I heard that endometriosis is not curable. It can continue to grow in severity and in another pelvic location. Female hormones, estrogen and progesterone, which are often prescribed to endometriosis sufferers, also exacerbate these feisty implants. It is like fertilizing a garden. The treatment promotes the disorder.

For years I had oscillated between excitement and fear at what could be the source of my constant pain. I decided to undergo the laparoscopy.

Surgery was easy. My medical team gave me a yummy drug delivered via I.V. before I was wheeled into the operating room. I felt woozy and euphoric. The next conscious thought I had was in the recovery room. I had an awful pain in my abdomen, and I didn't know whether to cry or throw up. I opted to cry, and the recovery room staff was all too ready to make me feel comfortable.

When I was strong enough to leave the recovery room, I returned to my room; my parents and sister were waiting. I looked for the doctor. Where was he? Was he right? Why wasn't he here? My mother gently told me that the doctor had his findings: endometriosis.

From that day, Nov. 11, 1987, I have gone through hell.

I have discovered what it means to hurt until you think you are going to pass out or die. I have discovered fear and complete abandonment. I have also discovered a faith in the field of medicine and the doctors who practice it.

I lived for years on addictive pain medicines only to be rewarded with more surgeries. After seven surgeries, I regained control by my decision, against my doctors' advice, for a complete hysterectomy. I was 27.

Losing my fertility as a young woman does not make me bitter. Ten years of surgeries, drug addiction, instability, lack of self-esteem, pain, suffering, indifference and ignorance does. One doctor actually told me to "buck up."

I will not let that happen to you. Here is a book that will answer your questions honestly, without judgment or patronizing tones. It will introduce you to many personal stories, culled from those of several thousand women I have connected with through our shared experiences. It will let you know what's waiting for you, whether you suspect you have endometriosis, have been recently diagnosed or have lived with pain most of your life. This book is to inform, comfort and affirm you. You are not alone.

" The tragedy of life is not so much what women suffer but what they miss."
—Anonymous

~CHAPTER ONE~

A CLOSER LOOK

MYTHS ABOUT ENDOMETRIOSIS

——— ◊ ———

Misdiagnosis is common among women who later learn they
have endometriosis

——— ◊ ———

The tragedy is, in large part, because of myths and misconceptions surrounding the disease and the women who have it.

Do any of these comments sound familiar?

~ "You are too young to have endometriosis."

~ "You are too old to have endometriosis"

~ "You can't have endometriosis; you've already had a hysterectomy."

~ "You have a sexually transmitted disease...we just can't find it yet!"

~ "You can't be in *that* much pain; you must be disproportionately describing the pain."

~ "You may be overworked or stressed; is your personal life O.K.?"

~ "Have you thought about seeing a psychotherapist?"

Angry? You bet. It's a crime that myths and ignorance can negatively impact so many woman who could otherwise be treated.

MISCONCEPTIONS

Doctors used to call endometriosis the "career woman's disease." This is because women who put off pregnancy were more likely to suffer from the disease in varying levels of severity. It was also once thought that endometriosis afflicted only white women as well as women who delayed childbearing.

———— ◊ ————

**Endometriosis does not discriminate.
It afflicts women of all races and ages.**

———— ◊ ————

Another myth that misleads many people is that women who have had hysterectomies cannot get endometriosis. Endometriosis may be located on *areas* other than the reproductive organs. I had endometriosis on my bowel, rectum and colon as well as the area between my bladder and vaginal wall. Some of it has come back. Hormone replacement therapy following hysterectomy may also aggravate dormant or microscopic endo implants overlooked in surgery or in areas that are simply "unremovable" (such as the colon and rectum).

Endometriosis can recur after surgical menopause or natural menopause. Microscopic cells on the bowel, bladder or other areas make the body still vulnerable to the disease. It happened to me and it can happen to you.

———— ◊ ————

**Without a doubt, the most crippling assumption is that
endometriosis is not a serious disease because it is not a killer.**

———— ◊ ————

But endometriosis is disabling and can destroy every aspect of a woman's life. It can savagely ruin relationships and careers. Severe depression and despondence can result in emotional and financial instability. A woman with endometriosis is constantly besieged by the conflict of pain and endurance. Any of these factors can grow in severity as the disease progresses and, without help, it can be overwhelming.

Stressful days at work or at home neither aggravate nor mitigate endometriosis pain. The pain is not in your head. The pain is very real and deserves to be seen and treated as such.

The last thing you need to fight, on top of the disease, is ignorance or misguided help. This book contains solid facts that will dispel false assumptions and help you, and those you love, to better understand what you're going through.

WHAT IS ENDOMETRIOSIS?

The word "endometriosis" comes from the Latin word *endometrium*, the tissue lining the uterus that builds up and is shed each month during a menstrual cycle. With endometriosis, tissue-like endometrium is found outside the uterus, on other areas of the abdomen and sometimes other parts of the body. These develop into what are called nodules, tumors, implants or growths. These, in turn, can cause pain, infertility and other problems.

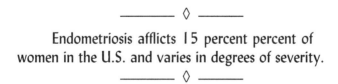

——— ◊ ———

Endometriosis afflicts 15 percent percent of women in the U.S. and varies in degrees of severity.

——— ◊ ———

Endometriosis can be extremely painful all the time and usually worsens around menstruation.

The most common location of endometrial implants is in the abdomen. This includes, but is not confined to, the ligaments supporting the uterus, the area between the vagina and the rectum, or the outer surface of the uterus and lining of the pelvic cavity. Diseased growths are also commonly found on the Fallopian tubes and ovaries. Rarely, there are growths found outside the abdomen, in the leg, lungs or another area.

The problem is this: Unlike the lining of the uterus, endometrial tissue outside the uterus has no way of leaving the body This results in internal bleeding, inflammation and formation of scar tissue. Usually, these implants are benign, but if left alone, will become more severe.

———— ◊ ————

A woman with endometriosis should have
continual care from her gynecologist

———— ◊ ————

WHAT DOES ENDOMETRIOSIS LOOK LIKE?

Relatively young implants look like pimples or clear blisters. Benign cysts called endometriomas may form on the ovaries. Many times these cysts are referred to as "chocolate cysts" because of the color of the old blood encapsulated within the cyst. Endometriomas can vary from pea-sized to larger than an orange.

Endometriosis can also appear web-like. Such adhesions can cover the uterus, tubes, ovaries and other surrounding regions. The webbing, visible under the laparoscope, resembles a spider web. The diseased implants may also look like burnt or decayed patches. This discoloration is the result of leftover blood and scar tissue.

WHAT CAUSES ENDOMETRIOSIS?

There is much speculation over the cause of endometriosis. One theory is that retrograde menstruation is responsible for menstrual tissue backing up through the Fallopian tubes, then settling in the abdominal cavity and growing. Another theory is that the lymph system is responsible for the distribution of endometrial tissue throughout the blood stream. Still another theory suggests genetic factors in which endometriosis may be carried in the genes.

It is not clear if elevated levels of cytokines in the peritoneal fluid lead to the development of endometriosis in women. Cytokines are components of the immune system that play a part in its maintenance. Peritoneal fluid is a naturally occurring fluid found in the abdomen. New theories arise as the medical profession learns more about the disease.

WHAT ARE THE SYMPTOMS?

If you don't know if you have endometriosis, don't hesitate to call your gynecologist to discuss it. The presence of abdominal pain, excessive or intermittent bleeding, shooting pains in your groin or abdomen, painful intercourse or painful bowel movements and urination signals a problem. Symptoms vary, but the most common are pain during and just before menstruation and during or after intercourse, irregular bleeding and difficulty conceiving.

Because diseases of the endometrium can exist simultaneously, the diagnostic process must rule out, as well as hone in on, specific diseases.

Blood levels may be taken to rule out anemia, diabetes and other systemic disorders. Blood can also be used to define your reproductive endocrine levels of FSH (follicle stimulating hormone) and estrogen. This is discussed in more detail later in the book.

The doctor will manually palpitate your uterus, cervix, ovaries and breasts as well as visually check, with the help of a speculum, your cervix and vagina. A Pap test should also be performed to evaluate your cervical health and to look for signs of dysplasia, abnormal cervical cells.

If a physical examination leaves the doctor with questions, a routine laparoscopy, D&C or endometrial biopsy may be necessary. Depending on the location of endometrial lesions, pain may also be experienced with bowel movements or strain. A little blood on the toilet tissue paper after a bowel movement may indicate endometrial implants on the rectum or bowel.

Amazingly, some women with the most severe endometriosis experience little or no pain and do not learn they have the disease until they find themselves unable to conceive. Infertility can effect approximately 40 percent of women with the disease.

———— ◊ ————

As the disease progresses without treatment, or sometimes even with, the chances of infertility increase.

———— ◊ ————

Another baffling aspect of endometriosis is that the amount of pain experienced is not correlated with the severity of the disease. Women with little or moderate endometriosis can experience debilitating pain while others with severe endometriosis experience little or no pain. This is one of the many reasons why endometriosis is so difficult to treat. This is also why a woman should be comfortable with and knowledgeable about her own body. In this way, changes can be detected and identified.

"Staging" endometriosis is a method some physicians use to determine the severity of the disease. The stages are one through five, with one being the mildest case of endometriosis and five being the most severe. Staging can present a problem as women with severe endometrial scarring may not feel much, if any, pain and women with stage one endometriosis may have crippling pain. I prefer using both a laparoscopy and the woman's personal pain as a correct diagnostic measure to the severity of her disease.

———— ◊ ————

Every woman has an obligation to know her body and how it functions.

———— ◊ ————

The information in this book will help you compile your ammunition when discussing your case with doctors.

IS THERE A CURE?

Unfortunately, there are no guaranteed medical techniques that make endometriosis disappear. The options for treatment are often a choice of the lesser of several evils. The course a woman takes depends on the woman herself, how she feels about her fertility needs and the severity of the illness. Severe endometriosis may be almost cured *only* with a radical hysterectomy, and even then endometriosis can return. Most otherwise healthy young women with their lives ahead of them do not wish this treatment.

A less drastic surgical treatment can include a laparoscopy, which excises current lesions but does not prevent new ones or a recurrence of the disease in new locations.

Another option is hormonal treatment, in which a woman's body is temporarily placed in "pseudo" pregnancy with continual birth-control pills, or "pseudo" menopause, with the intent to decrease or cease production of the two big fertilizers for endometriosis, estrogen and progesterone. As with natural menopause, annoying to severely debilitating side effects can emerge, ranging from hot flashes to complete cessation of menstruation.

A major drawback to the "maintenance" strategy of treating endometriosis is the possibility of narcotic drug addiction. Pain medications are often prescribed to combat the discomfort, making addiction a very real concern. I became addicted to narcotic pain relievers and tranquilizers, as well as to sleeping pills—anything to avoid the pain. I wanted more and more to escape rather than to learn to tolerate the intense discomfort.

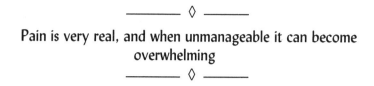

Pain is very real, and when unmanageable it can become
overwhelming

After being alone with my torture for long periods of time, all I wanted to do was shrink into a little speck and disappear. I became depressed and isolated from everyone and everything, except my prescription bottles. Numbness is where I wanted to be but where I *never, ever* want to be again.

I no longer use pain medications as a physical or emotional release. Reaching this level took a lot of hard work and support, and I am still unsure if I would have retrieved my sanity had I not had a hysterectomy. The cycle of pain was so powerful, I probably would have spiraled deeper into a pit of despair.

Not all doctors freely and easily dispense medications, and I do not wish to discredit the entire medical community nor the importance of managing severe pain. But I would like to provide you with more options to handle pain, including non-medicinal practices such as support groups, learning centers and public forums.

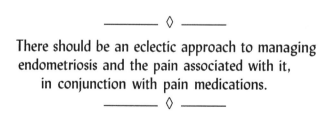

There should be an eclectic approach to managing
endometriosis and the pain associated with it,
in conjunction with pain medications.

Because endometriosis is recurring and difficult to excise altogether, it can be frustrating for women to deal with. The disease is as unique as the person it invades, and because there are degrees of endometriosis, women must be exposed to *all* information and all possible strategies, from the least invasive to a definitive surgery.

I had to fight all the way to the operating room to get my hysterectomy, and that was after seven surgeries. I do not wish for any other woman to have to endure the years of pain that I might have avoided if only my endometriosis had been treated earlier and more aggressively. I understand that in the beginning keeping my fertility intact was a major concern, but when the pain and suffering interfered with my work, my relationships and my life in general, it was time to rethink my priorities.

ENDOMETRIOSIS ON THE BOWEL & BLADDER

Women with endometriosis can experience intestinal symptoms such as constipation, bloody stools, pain with strain or bowel movements, and diarrhea. This can be attributed to adhesions in the intestines or overproduction of specific prostaglandins.

Because the symptoms mimic other intestinal disorders, endometriosis is often overlooked as a diagnosis, especially if a woman is young or has children. Often, endometriosis on the bowel is left untouched and pain and bowel problems may persist despite total hysterectomy, hormonal therapies and excision of all other pelvic lesions.

Before you walk out of the doctor's office with these symptoms, make it clear that you want to know how such symptoms *might* be related to endometriosis on your rectum, colon or bladder.

I had a significant amount of endometriosis on and around my rectum and colon and was told for years to take Metamucil for what was thought to be irritable bowel syndrome. It was only after I put pressure on the doctor to do another laparoscopy that he found endometriosis in the exact areas that were causing my pain and discomfort: my colon and rectum.

——— ◊ ———

Your body is sending signals;
find someone who will listen to you

——— ◊ ———

Having endometriosis on the bladder can be extremely painful and difficult both to diagnose and treat. You may experience pain and discomfort with a full bladder, or have difficulty voiding. The reason endometriosis is so difficult to treat surgically in these areas is because damage to the rectum, colon or bladder can be serious and permanent. These are vital organs and oftentimes physicians would rather leave the growths that have adhered to these areas than cauterize or excise them for fear of perforation. This is when you may be placed on Lupron, Danazol, Synarel or another hormonal drug to help shrink the growths.

ADHESIONS

One of the many complications that can arise from endometriosis is the formation of adhesions. These masses can bind to or block areas, resulting in infertility and increased pain and sometimes even requiring surgery. I had seven laparoscopies and a total hysterectomy before I found out how devastating adhesions can be.

I woke up with a severe stomachache on a Monday morning, seven months after my hysterectomy, and the next thing I knew I was having emergency surgery because of a bowel obstruction caused by adhesions.

This sounds like a vicious cycle, doesn't it? If you need surgery to remove the endometriosis, you invariably leave behind scar tissue that may form into adhesions. Often a woman will have to have additional surgeries to remove adhesions formed from her previous surgeries to remove the endometriosis.

The most common sites for adhesions are pelvic organs. They can also form over the endometriosis implants themselves. The most predominant sites for adhesions are on the bowels. These can invite a host of other symptoms and illnesses in a class of their own. Symptoms include pain, nausea, intestinal blockage and irritable bowel syndrome, to name a few. If you have a bowel obstruction, you may experience a sharp stabbing or squeezing pain in your stomach as well as projectile vomiting that appears green or brown accompanied by an awful stench. You may also experience a high fever of 101-plus degrees. Any of these symptoms should be checked out by a doctor immediately. The doctor will want to do an abdominal X-ray series to see if and where your blockage exists.

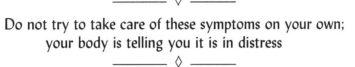

Do not try to take care of these symptoms on your own;
your body is telling you it is in distress

Several treatments are being explored that can be used during surgery to prevent the formation of adhesions, but adhesion formation remains one of the major silent, long-term side effects of multiple surgeries for endometriosis.

ENDOMETRIOSIS & INFERTILITY

Endometriosis is an evident cause of infertility.

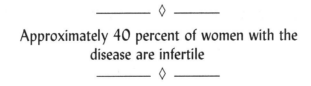

Approximately 40 percent of women with the
disease are infertile

The likelihood for ectopic pregnancies and mis-carriages is significantly higher in women with endometriosis than in others. Even relatively slight cases of endometriosis can render a woman infertile. Many factors contribute to a woman's infertility. In laboratory animals, it is shown those surgically inducted with endometriosis experience a decrease in fertility from 70 percent to 30 percent.

Endometriosis also affects the peritoneal environment which can also cause infertility. The peritoneum covers the surface of the uterus, parts of the intestines and other structures inside the abdomen and pelvis. With endometriosis there is an increased amount of peritoneal fluid. Scavenger white blood cells begin to lose their capacity to clear away disease. This can affect sperm interaction, mobility and survival. Also, during menstruation, blood may drip from the Fallopian tubes and irritate the peritoneum, causing swelling. Bleeding from the Fallopian tubes is called retrograde menstruation.

With women who have "severe pelvic regions," in which the ovary is encapsulated, may also have the condition described as luteinized unruptured follicle (LUF). This occurs when the egg is not released from the ovary. Endometriosis is found in roughly 60 percent of those with LUF. Women with ovulatory dysfunction may experience infertility. It has also been noted that the immune system is affected by endometriosis and this can negatively affect fertility.

PREGNANCY

Surgery may "buy time" for a woman who wants children; however, surgery does not effectively cure endometriosis; as a result, its recurrence is likely. Pregnancy frequently offers a temporary reprieve from symptoms. Many women opt for multiple surgeries, conservatively done.

Pregnancy rates after conservative surgery vary depending on the severity of the disease. They generally range from 55 percent to 60 percent for those with moderate endometriosis. It is believed that infertility is more of a problem in women who have had the disease for a long time.

———— ◊ ————

Many women with the disease are urged to have
children as soon as possible; chances for pregnancy
decline as the disease progresses.

———— ◊ ————

HOW ARE RELATIONSHIPS AFFECTED?

When a woman is suffering debilitating cramping
and/or stabbing pain, sexual thoughts are on a far-distant
planet. I did not want to be touched, let alone have
intercourse, and that created rifts that caused even the
strongest of relationships to suffer.

Endometriosis also wreaks havoc on finances. There
are days or weeks each year when you're in too much pain
to go to work and, for many, that significantly alters
household income. There are medical costs of surgeries,
pain medications, hormonal medications and other drugs,
as well as doctors' appointments and laboratory tests,
ultrasound, sonogram, MRI, CT scan and other
procedures your physician may order. Depending on the
choice of therapy, monthly costs for hormonal
medications to control endometriosis can range from $100
to $600. A laparoscopy could cost $10,000 to $20,000,
depending on the procedure and medications given
during the surgery.

While these may be effective measures in controlling
symptoms, medications and laparoscopies are just a
measure of maintenance. Usually a woman who is
afflicted with endometriosis at an early age, such as
myself, will have two to six surgeries before opting for a
hysterectomy.

As if preparing, enduring and recovering from
surgeries were not enough, there is also the well-known
"biological clock" pressures. I was told that getting
pregnant would help my endometriosis and possibly be
my only chance to conceive—but at the time I was a single
college student and pregnancy was not a realistic option.
Through three relationships I waited for a proposal of
marriage so I could get pregnant, have at least one child,

and then finally view a hysterectomy more favorably. I began looking at men as sperm-makers rather than as quality people, one of whom might eventually be "Mr. Right." My relationships were jeopardized by my constant dilemma: to have or not to have a hysterectomy.

———— ◊ ————

**I was scared of letting down my doctors,
my family and, most of all, myself**

———— ◊ ————

How could I possibly desecrate all my femininity by having my uterus—my "baby maker"—taken from me? So I remained a trouper, but to whom? Certainly not to myself.

HOW ELSE ARE YOU AFFECTED?

As the years passed without a resolution, I began to live with pain as an expected part of my life. Friends and family became accustomed to my woes and my inability to participate in many of the joys of life. The cruelest trick of all is that there were moments of total clarity and strength, at which times I would march to my gynecologist and *show* him (and the others) that I was going to buck up and deal with my fate as an adult. These moments were quickly smothered by another episode of unbearable pain, at which I would scream for a hysterectomy.

Various of my doctors made it clear they thought I was nuts. One doctor wrote chastising remarks in my medical records implying that I was "faking it." I am no longer under his care.

Not only did I feel upset and frustrated at these peaks and troughs, but also embarrassed and humiliated at the prospect of my gynecologist documenting his disbelief. This is in my medical record, the one that gets passed around the HMO I participate in. I could picture all the doctors around a big round table reading and laughing at it. Laughing at me. At times it seemed like such a "boys club."

It was a woman oncologist/gynecologist who recommended a hysterectomy—while questioning why I hadn't had one. Looking back at my long trail of surgeries with high doses of Lupron, birth-control pills and pain medications, she was surprised that I had not considered a hysterectomy earlier. I had considered it several times, only to be put off by my former gynecologist or reminded of my fickle feelings. I came to see that she was a sincere and kind physician. I walked into her office with a plan for sustenance and walked out with a plan for my life.

I have such gratitude for the two gynecologists who took a chance and gave me back my life. I finally felt I had encountered truth and with it the easing of an enormous burden. Two doctors heard my pain, touched my pain and wanted to end my pain. I will forever be grateful.

For so long I had felt the weight of being both patient and doctor, player and coach, teacher and student. It had been ten years of what finally had seemed fruitless hours of research and options .

I had to learn to be my own health advocate. In the process, I learned to sail against the prevailing winds of medical opinion and arrogance and to really believe in myself through learning to know my own body. In essence, my womanhood emerged as a result of the hysterectomy. Instead of feeling bereft, I felt stronger than ever.

I still had surgical pain a week after surgery, but none of the debilitating and severe endometriosis pain I had up to the minute of surgery. I am free of the bondage my pain brought forth. I feel a sense of renewal and hope that I had only previously dreamed of.

Women with endometriosis are finally becoming strong enough to express their anger and frustration. I hope I can speak for those who do not yet feel the strength and resolve necessary to deal effectively with this disease, even though it will come soon enough.

I want to force the medical profession to take this affliction seriously, to fund research that can lead to real understanding of this disease. Women suffer immensely, and the medical community's frequent way of dealing with women who present these confusing symptoms—placating them rather than taking their complaints seriously—is not the safest game to play.

Psychological factors can be equally debilitating for women with endometriosis and are compounded when they are treated dismissively. Women should not be afraid of or intimidated by their physicians. If you feel you are not being heard, even for one moment, change doctors. Working together, we can accomplish miracles, and every woman deserves a miracle or two.

MAKING YOUR VOCABULARY "DOCTOR FRIENDLY"

Before we're hit with the diagnosis we're bombarded with medical jargon that would confuse a pre-med student. That's O.K. Here are explanations of words that soon will be all too familiar to you.

Abdomen—Part of the body that contains the stomach, small intestine, colon, rectum, liver, spleen, pancreas, gallbladder and bladder.

Abscess—Local accumulation of pus anywhere in the body.

Acupressure—Pressure on set points of the body to relieve pain.

Acupuncture—Insertion of needles on specific areas of the body to relieve pain.

Adhesion—Scar-tissue strands that can form in an area of a previous operation, such as a laparoscopy or laparotomy.

Advocacy—Ensuring optimal, high-quality health care, using your own voice.

Amino acids—Organic compound for forming peptides.

Analgesic—Something given to relieve pain.

Analog—Drug compound that acts like another substance, but with different effects.

Androgen—A hormone that promotes the development and maintenance of male sex characteristics.

Anesthesia—Loss of feeling of awareness. A local anesthetic causes loss of feeling in a part of the body. A general anesthetic puts the person to sleep.

Anus—The opening of the rectum to the outside of the body.

Appendectomy—Removal of the appendix.

Atrophy—To shrink.

Benign—Non-cancerous.

Beta endorphins—Naturally occurring "happy hormones."

Biopsy—The removal of a sample of tissue for examination under a microscope to check for cancer or other cells.

Birth-control pills—Method used to control menstruation and pain. Also used as contraceptive.

Bladder—The organ that stores urine.

Bone density—The amount of bone tissue in a specific volume of bone.

Bowel—Another name for the intestines, which consist of a large and a small bowel.

Bowel obstruction—Blockage that causes failure of intestinal contents to pass through bowel.

Bowel prep—Preparation to clear the bowel of stool prior to surgery.

Calcium—A mineral mainly found in the hard part of the bones. Bones store calcium.

CAT scan—Computerized Axial Tomography.

Catheter—Any hollow, flexible tubing inserted into the body to add or remove fluids.

Cancer—Abnormal cell growth.

Cauterization—The use of heat to destroy abnormal cells.

Cervix—The neck of an organ, such as the uterus.

Chocolate cysts—Endometriosis implants or cysts filled with old blood.

Colon—Long, coiled, tube-like organ that removes water from digested food. The remaining material, called stool, leaves the body via the anus. The colon is sometimes referred to as the large bowel or large intestine.

Colonoscopy—A viewing tube inserted into the rectum to inspect the colon.

Colposcopy—A lighted magnifying instrument used to examine the vagina and cervix.

Cul-de-sac—Pouch at the base of the abdominal cavity.

Cyst—Fluid filled sac.

Cytokines—Interferes with implantation of embryo.

Danazol—Drug commonly used to treat endometriosis. A Gonadotropin inhibitor.

Depo-Provera -The drug that causes cessation of progesterone and estrogen.

Depression—Low spirits, loss of self-worth, apathy, withdrawal and fatigue.

Diaphragm—Dome-shaped muscle that separates chest cavity from abdominal cavity. Aids in breathing.

Dilatation and Curettage (D&C)—Operation in which the cervix is expanded enough to permit cervical canal and uterine lining to be scraped with a curette.

Dyspareunia—Pain during sexual intercourse.

Dysmenorrhea—Pain associated with menstruation.

Endometrioma—A tumor containing endometrial tissue.

Endometriosis—Disease where endometrial tissue grows outside the endometrium, often in other parts of the abdomen.

Endometrium—Inner layer on the uterus.

Estrogen—Female hormone produced by the ovaries.

Fallopian Tubes—Tubes on each side of the uterus that convey the egg from the ovary to the uterus.

FDA—Federal Drug Administration.

Fertilization—Process of combining the male gamete with the female ovum, resulting in a zygote.

Fibroid—A benign uterine tumor.

Follicle Stimulating Hormone—Pituitary hormone that stimulates follicle growth in women and sperm formation in men.

Gland—Organ that produces and secretes body fluids or substances, such as hormones.

Homeopathy—System of healing based on the theory that, "like heals like."

GnRH—Hormone produced and released by the hypothalamus that controls the pituitary gland's production and release of gonadotropins.

Hormone Replacement Therapy (HRT)—Replacements of estrogens and progestins after surgical or natural menopause.

Hormones—Chemicals produced by endocrine glands to regulate various body functions.

Hysterectomy—Surgical removal of the uterus.

Hysteroscopy—Outpatient procedure to inspect the inside of the uterus.

Infertility—Inability to conceive.

Insomnia—Chronic inability to sleep.

I.V.—Inside a vein, also call intravenous.

I.V.F.—In Vitro Fertilization.

Laparoscopy—Exploratory abdominal surgery to view the inside of the abdomen for endometriosis or other problems.

Laparotomy—Surgical procedure reserved for severe cases of endometriosis.

Laser—A powerful beam of pure light used in some types of surgery to cut or destroy tissue.

Lesion—An area of abnormal tissue damage.

LUNA—Surgical technique where uterosacral nerves and ligaments are severed.

Lupron—GnRh or gonadotropin releasing hormone.

Luteinizing—Hormone-releasing hormone (GnRh) Hormone that controls sex hormones in men and women.

Menopause—The gradual or surgical cessation of menstruation.

MRI—Magnetic resonance Imagery.

Myomectomy—Surgical removal of a uterine fibroid tumor.

Nausea—Feeling of abdominal sickness with urge to vomit.

Nerve—A bundle of fibers that uses electrical and chemical signals to transmit sensory and motor information from one body part to another.

Norplant—A proprietary contraceptive measure.

NSAIDS—Non-Steroid Anti-Inflammatory Drugs used for pain management.

OB-GYN—Physician specializing in female reproductive disorders and pregnancy.

Ombudsman—A person who acts as liaison between patient and health care providers.

Oophorectomy—Surgical removal of the ovaries.

Operative report—Written report about the events occurring during your surgery.

Opiates—Narcotic pain medicines.

Ovary—Gonadal gland in the female that produces eggs(ova) for reproduction and the two female sex hormones, estrogen and progesterone.

Ovulation—Monthly ripening and discharging of an egg (ovum) from the ovary. It occurs approximately fourteen days before the onset of a menstrual period.

PAP Test—Microscopic examination of cells collected from cervix.

Pathology—Study of cause and effects of disease.

Peritoneum—The tissue layer of cells lining the inner wall of the abdomen and pelvis.

Polyp—A mass of tissue that develops on inside wall of a hollow organ, such as the colon.

Presacral neurectomy—Interruption of the pain fibers nearest to the lowest vertebrae.

Prosteglandins—Hormone-like chemicals that variously affect the reproductive organs.

Progesterone—Female sex hormone responsible for, among other things, the thickening of the uterine lining before conception.

QI—Chinese concept of energy.

Rectum—Last 6 to 8 inches of the large intestine.

Recur—To occur again.

Reproductive system—The organs directly involved with producing eggs and in conceiving and carrying babies.

Retrograde menstruation—Backward flow of blood during menstruation.

Retroverted uterus—Tilted uterus.

Salpingo—Oophorectomy—Surgical removal of ovaries and Fallopian tubes.

Seprecur—GnRH analog.

Spastic colon—Irritable Bowel Syndrome.

Speculum—Instrument used to widen the opening of the vagina so the cervix is more easily visible.

Steroids—Large number of hormone-like substances.

Surgery—An operation.

Synarel—GnRH analog.

Testosterone—A male sex hormone.

Trigonitus—Disorder of the bladder.

Tubal Ligation—Sterilization process that blocks both Fallopian tubes.

Tumor—An abnormal mass of tissue.

Ultrasound (Sonography)—A test where high frequency sound waves are bounced off tissues and the echoes are converted into a picture.

Ureters—Tubes that carry urine from each kidney to the bladder.

Urologist—A physician who specializes in disorders of the urinary organs.

Uterus—A small, pear shaped muscular organ in the pelvis of females where the unborn child develops until birth. Also called the womb.

Vagina—Tube of muscle and membrane connecting the external female genitalia with the uterus.

Vaginitus—Swelling or infection of vaginal tissue.

Visualization—Self-guided imagery used to soothe pain.

Western Medicine—Traditional medicinal practices.

X-ray—High energy radiation.

Yeast Infection—Fungal Infection. Also called Candida.

Zoladex—GnRh agonist.

~

Chapter Two

What's Best For You?

You're looking for straight information that will help you make an intelligent decision about your body.

———— ◊ ————

Your decision will impact your life forever.

———— ◊ ————

After years of doing research, consulting experts and listening to women who have faced this same quandary, I have compiled this section of various treatments—from holistic to surgical.

Your medical team should be consulted while you are mulling over your decision. This chapter is certainly not meant to replace your physician's advice but, rather, to offer supplemental alternatives.

Before you decide on treatment, it's important to understand your theraputic goal. You may fall into one of these five categories:

1.   Women of reproductive age who do not desire pregnancy at this time but want their fertility intact.

2.   Women of reproductive age, already infertile, but who would like to keep their uterus so they can later become impregnated through In-Vitro Fertilization (IVF).

3.   Women with recurrent symptoms after all options have been exhausted, but who still want their fertility to remain intact.

4.   Women for whom childbearing is either completed or not a priority.

5.   Women who have had a hysterectomy.

Like me, some of you may not fit neatly into a specific category. Maybe you are a little of everything. Through my years of dealing with endometriosis, my priorities, wants and needs changed dramatically.

HOMEOPATHY

Women around the world have managed their endometriosis with homeopathic treatments.

Homeopathy is a school of medicine based on the belief that humans have the ability to heal themselves. Homeopathic remedies stimulate this ability and empower the body's healing capabilities. The remedy reinforces the healing process by working with, as opposed to against, the body. For example, if a woman is suffering from Dysmenorrhea, she would take the herb, "cocculus indicus," which stimulates her symptoms of cramping, dizziness and weakness.

The word "homeopathy" comes from the Greek word "homoios," which means like, and "pathos," which means suffering. It is based on the law of similars: A substance that creates a symptom in an otherwise healthy individual can treat that same symptom in an ill person.

Western medicines attempt to destroy bad cells associated with the disease or suppress the symptoms that accompany it. This process may require strong synthetic drugs that attack the body. This, in turn, can create annoying to potentially dangerous side effects. Homeopathic medicines work with, as opposed to against, the body's natural ability to heal itself. There are also few, if any, side effects created by homeopathic remedies, although their effects have not been documented as closely as FDA-approved medications. The absence of side effects is especially crucial for those who have difficulty tolerating the effects of synthetic drugs. Homeopathic remedies can be found at most health food stores.

Homeopathic pills or pellets can be taken sublingually—placed under the tongue—which allows enough time for the medication to absorb into the mucus membranes and into the bloodstream. There is no metabolizing done by the stomach, as with traditional medicines, this alleviates stress on your kidneys, liver and esophageal lining.

Here are common homeopathic medicines and the symptoms they combat. The remedy to use is the one that elicits symptoms most similar to the ones you are experiencing.

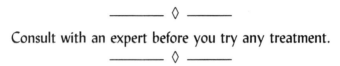

Consult with an expert before you try any treatment.

Not everyone can achieve marked pain relief from homeopathic medication; I certainly could not for severe endometriosis pain, but many women swear by it—and more power to them! It is worth a try!

PMS
~ Lachesis mutus: eases menstrual pain, which can be worse after sleep or with heat.
~ Lycopodium clavatum: irritability; apprehension; aggressiveness.
~ Nux vomica: irritability; chills; spasms.
~ Sepia: anxiety; sadness; fear; indifference; chills.

Dysmenorrhea
~ Cocculus indicus: Crampy pains; dizziness; weakness.
~ Sepia: Menstrual pain; irregular menses; chills.
~ Sabina: Pain in lower back or abdomen.
~ Pulsatilla: Irregular flow; pain; restlessness; condition improves with fresh air.
~ Magnesia phosphorica: Spasmodic pain; condition improves with warmth.

Menopause
~ Sepia: Hot flashes with chills or sweats; fatigue.
~ Lachesis mutus: Hot flashes; headache; condition worsens with heat.

Acupuncture & Acupressure

Acupuncture is the insertion of very fine needles to stimulate certain points on the body's surface. This influences the physiological functioning of the body as a whole as well as specific parts. Heat produced by burning herbs or "moxibustion," the application of light pressure through acupressure; and massage and exercise, may also be included.

This is based on the Chinese concept of QI (pronounced key). This roughly translates to "energy." QI is the life force within us. It encompasses all vital activity, including spiritual, emotional, mental and physical. We are influenced by the flow of QI within our bodies. This can be disrupted by internal or external factors, and when QI is blocked, we fall ill. As with "yin" and "yang," when there isn't a balance, we and the things around us do not work smoothly.

Achieving balance means getting all aspects of our lives to run smoothly and effectively. This includes work, family, and self. Our energy can be skewed by the least imbalance.

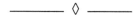

It is up to us to be so spiritually aligned with ourselves that we are able to notice and remedy such a situation.

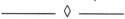

These alternative methods offer different approaches you can use in conjunction with necessary surgery or medicinal treatment. Again, results vary, as each woman presents a different case history and persona.

Just as NSAIDS (Non-Steroidal Anti-Inflammatory Drugs) help to relax the muscles of the body, so does acupressure. In some instances, I really think it helps when used in conjunction *with* medications. Many women use acupuncture and acupressure when they feel cramping tightness in their bodies. These are effective ways to reduce tightness and help the body to relax. This in itself can reduce pain.

Relaxation is difficult to achieve when you are experiencing pain, I know! It is frustrating when people say, "Just relax and take a deep breath." It is at that point I usually want to hit something or someone. When I was in a great deal of pain, I was tense. How could I achieve a relaxed state when the pain was relentless? I was frustrated.

It was my therapist who helped me discover these tools of acupuncture and acupressure to achieve a relaxed enough state where I could at least *try* to imagine myself serene.

There were times where I did not want to be touched at all. It was as if my skin were hypersensitive. If you can stand being touched, massage is an excellent way to help your body unwind and relax. This feels especially good on your lower back and shoulders. There are also pressure points in your feet and hands that correspond to specific parts of the body. Stimulating these areas often provides relief from tension. Massaging the area in between the thumb and index finger (right below the webbing in the muscle) is said to provide relief from tension headaches.

Wouldn't it be nice if medical science could come up with a spot on our body we could rub and all our endometriosis pain would go away? Maybe someday! For now, we must take it bit by bit and come up with a formula of relief unique for each of us. This can be discovered only through trial and error.

RELAXATION & VISUALIZATION TECHNIQUES

Pain is a very real physiological phenomenon. We know this all too well. Our body's ability (or lack of ability) to relax is intricately interwoven with our sensations of pain. Those with consistent pain need to learn to use relaxation and visualization to relieve muscle tension and tight spots. Pain leads to tension, which fatigues us, and then the pain kicks in again! Frustrating, but the good news is we can break the cycle.

———— ◊ ————

Relaxation and visualization are skills, and like any skills, they must be practiced regularly.

———— ◊ ————

Don't get frustrated if you do not feel complete pain relief after one or two sessions. Make small, attainable goals and reward yourself with each goal met. With endometriosis, many muscles are working overtime, expending precious energy and an increasing fatigue. Our bodies have been "programmed" to remain in a "fight or flight" state, preparing for its next battle with pain. We are in constant state of agitation, and we do not realize how tense we have become. Here are three steps that will get you started on relaxing both your body and mind:

1. Begin to recognize body tension vs. a relaxed state. Note the difference. Learn to keep your shoulders relaxed and in alignment.

2. Maintain good posture at all times, including when walking, standing, sitting or stretching. Good posture takes less energy and gives all of your body better support.

3. Develop "effortless" breathing. Use the diaphragm (a large muscle below the rib cage and visible when we breathe) and breathe from your chest. Inhale and exhale for the same length of time. When we are tense or in pain, we tend to have rapid, shallow breathing; it is our bodies' natural reaction to stress (and pain is extremely stressful).

———— ◊ ————

Deep breathing is the easiest way to begin relaxing.

———— ◊ ————

Here are some tips for inhaling and exhaling:

Inhale: Sit, stand, or lie on a flat surface. Place your hands gently on your stomach and inhale through your nose, letting your stomach expand. Feel the rise with your hands.

Exhale: Keeping your hands on your stomach, exhale slowly through your mouth, controlling the speed of your exhalation. Your stomach will deflate while your diaphragm contracts.

When your lungs feel empty, repeat the process. Do this three or four times at an easy pace. By placing the hands on the stomach, we can feel if we are breathing properly. If our stomachs tighten when we breathe in we know we are doing this incorrectly.

Another technique is Progressive Muscle Relaxation, a three-step exercise. First you tense a muscle and notice how it feels, then release the tension and be aware of how this feels, then concentrate on comparing the two sensations, familiarizing yourself with their marked differences. Move to various other muscles on your body until you are completely relaxed.

Meditation is another terrific way to relax. It begins in a quiet environment with steady, tranquil breathing. The main objective is to clear the mind and concentrate on a single object, image or sound for an extended period.

Visualization and Guided Imagery are yet other excellent tools when we are in pain.

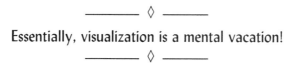

Essentially, visualization is a mental vacation!

Go there wherever you feel most serene and safe. Picture yourself relaxed and without pain. Guided imagery is usually combined with relaxation techniques to deepen concentration, maximize relaxation and extend the reprieve from pain or stress.

ANALGESICS

Pain is a very real part of endometriosis. Managing it, although necessary, has also become controversial. Because endometriosis is a progressive disease and has accompanying pain regardless of how severe the disease is, many women need prescription painkillers or analgesics to reduce the pain. But some pain medications can be addictive, with women needing ever-higher doses of the same medication to relieve the same pain. This is called tolerance and can happen even if you do not feel "addicted."

Aside from physiological addiction, there is psychological addiction.

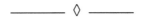

A woman can come to depend so completely on these narcotics that she will worry that they may be taken away.

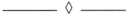

My pain medications were a coveted lot. I was constantly counting them and worrying that I would run out. If I did, which doctor would I telephone? And would he or she dispense more without asking too many questions?

This was my experience. Many women are able to fully control these substances, but there are many like me who cannot. I also know that many doctors are carefully involved with their patients' medications and do not allow triplicate copies of narcotic prescriptions to be made, while some are not. This is yet another reason to become your own educator and advocate. If you are worried about addiction, talk with your physician. If you feel unsatisfied with the answers you are given, talk with another health-care provider.

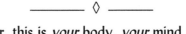

Remember, this is *your* body, *your* mind and *your* opportunity to have a say in *your* health care.

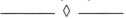

Pain medications are important to the suffering woman. I don't know what I would have done without some of them. Yet when a person remains on these medications for months or years, alternatives should be presented. If the pain is horrific, which it was for me, it's time to rethink your strategy. For many women, this is the hardest part—trying to decipher what to do and in which order and to what expense. Social, religious, personal and physician biases can strongly influence a decision that is truly only the woman's to make.

FREQUENTLY ASKED QUESTIONS ABOUT PAIN MANAGEMENT

1. *What are OTC medications?*

    OTC means "over the counter," or non-prescription, medications. These include aspirin and ibuprofen, medications that provide relief for mild pain associated with dysmenorrhea.

2. *What are prescription analgesics?*

    These are pain medications prescribed by a physician, usually for moderate to severe pain. There are several types of prescription analgesics, such as Vicodin, Tylenol with codeine or Darvocet.

3. *What are opiates or narcotic medications?*

    Opiates are pain medications derived from the opium poppy. These are usually prescribed for moderate to severe pain or for those who are no longer relieved by non-opiate medications. These include morphine, Demerol and fentanyl.

4. *What are alternative medical treatments?*

    These encompass a wide array of practices from homeopathic remedies to acupuncture and acupressure. Essentially, "alternative medicine" is a term used for non-Western medicine. These are focused on more natural antidotes, as opposed to synthetic remedies for pain.

5. *What are relaxation and visualization?*

    These are methods used to naturally relax the body and mind. They aim to create a state of calmness to help ease muscle tension and pain.

HORMONAL THERAPY

Hormonal treatment aims to induce atrophy or regression of endometrial implants or adhesions by relying on the absence of estrogen and progesterone. Unfortunately, this method is ineffective in advanced stages of endometriosis with excessive growths.

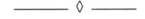

Hormonal therapy usually offers temporary relief, with symptoms recurring within one to two years, sometimes sooner.

Side effects range from unpleasant to ghastly, depending on the drug. Hormonal therapy is also expensive and thus not feasible for many women.

Choices of hormonal treatment include gonado-trophin releasing hormone agonists (GnRh). These induce a "pseudo" menopausal state, stopping menstruation and lowering levels of estrogen. Among these are Synarel, Lupron, Zoladex and Suprecur. Hormones such as these are used to treat both the symptoms and the disease by shrinking growths.

GnRh is a small hormone composed of ten amino acids; it controls the release of hormones from the anterior pituitary gland. The pituitary gland affects ovarian function. These therapies offer symptomatic relief that, again, varies among women. These drugs can be safely used only for up to six months because of loss in bone density and decreasing levels of calcium. Normal ovarian function resumes once the medication is discontinued.

Danazol is a synthetic testosterone derivative or synthetic progestin also prescribed to treat endometriosis. It is similar to the GnRh analogs in that it aims to decrease the production of estrogen and shrink lesions. Danazol has many androgenic side effects because it acts like the male hormone testosterone. These include acne, weight gain and reduction in breast size. Again, as with the GnRh agonists, once a woman is off the medication, normal ovarian function resumes and its side-effects usually, but not always, disappear.

There are other hormones available to treat endometriosis, such as the birth-control pills, Depo-provera and Norplant. These treat the symptoms but not the condition. These drugs mimic a state of pregnancy, postponing ovulation and the production of estrogen by the ovaries.

I was placed on Lupron twice, each time with a different effect. My first round of hormonal therapy proved successful for six months, and I had minimal side effects. When I began experiencing symptoms again and could no longer remain safely on Lupron, I opted for another laparoscopy. I did not want another surgery but could not tolerate the pain and discomfort.

This was my fifth surgery and I had a LUNA. This technique divides the uteral sacral ligaments and nerves that house the para-sympathetic and sympathetic nerves. This procedure is most helpful for women suffering from mid-line pain or dysmenorrhea and less effective in abating the pain induced by the endometrial implants themselves. This procedure provided me with a temporary respite from the severity of symptoms I had felt, but, within a year, I was experiencing pain to the levels of needing narcotic medication.

It was a vicious cycle. I was again placed on Lupron, and this time the effects were horrible. I had several hot flashes daily and felt lethargic and depressed. I gained weight and lost hope.

Perhaps the most frustrating aspect of endometriosis is that maintenance is all consuming if you don't opt for a hysterectomy. As I began to analyze my history, I slowly began thinking it was time to make a change. For the next year I relied heavily on narcotics and fell into a deep depression. I was bankrupt, both physically and emotionally, and I could not see any way out of the dark abyss.

FREQUENTLY ASKED QUESTIONS ABOUT MEDICAL/HORMONAL TREATMENT

1. *What role do oral contraceptives play?*

    Continued use of oral contraceptives places the body in a state of "pseudo" pregnancy, regulating hormone levels and the release of estrogen from the ovaries.

2. *What are GnRH medications, and what do they do?*

    GnRH analogs prevent the natural releasing hormones from being secreted, blocking their stimulating effect on the ovaries. The normal production of estrogen is reduced, and the body is placed into temporary menopause. GnRH analogs affect the hypothalamus and the pituitary gland and decrease leutinized hormone (LH) and follicle stimulated hormonc (FSH) secretion. Because endometriosis flourishes on estrogen, regression often occurs rapidly. These drugs aim to atrophy or shrink existing lesions and can be used safely for only six months. Lupron and Synarel are examples of GnRH analogs.

3. *What are the side effects of these medications?*

    Side effects of GnRH analogs include, but are not exclusive to, hot flashes, vaginal dryness, weight gain, reduction in breast size, mood swings, depression, headaches and interruption of normal sleep patterns. Again, this varies by patient.

4. *What are the long-term effects of these medications?*

    Unfortunately, this is inconclusive because these drugs are relatively new.

5. *Will this cure endometriosis?*

    No. There is no known cure for endometriosis. There is only maintenance through surgical and medicinal methods.

ADD-BACK THERAPY

Add-back therapy is when the doctor may prescribe hormone replacement in conjunction with a GnRH analog. This is to reduce some of the more harmful effects of taking the analogs, such as loss of bone density, and other uncomfortable side effects, such as hot flashes and vaginal dryness. It varies from woman to woman; what works for one may not for someone else.

There are two types of add-back therapy, hormonal and non-hormonal. Hormonal therapy combines GnRH analogs with sex steroids, such as estrogen and progesterone. Non-hormonal therapy includes use of calcitonin or phosphates, such as etidronate.

The optimum add-back therapy remains to be seen, however, studies indicate that add-back therapy prevents side effects associated with the use of GnRH agonists alone.

——— ◊ ———

Add-back therapy can also allow a woman to safely remain on agonists longer than the suggested six to nine months.

——— ◊ ———

ADJUNCTIVE THERAPY

Once a woman has exploratory surgery and it is evident that endometriosis is present, hormonal therapy may be used in addition to lengthen the relief of symptoms in some women. Which drug to use should be decided by the woman and her gynecologist.

I would imagine most women would want the most conservative method in treating endometriosis. This is especially true when fertility is an issue. There are many factors that play a part. I wanted to fight. For my fertility, my womanhood, my family ideals and values.

——— ◊ ———

What I wasn't fighting for was me.

——— ◊ ———

I compromised years of my life, accepting pain, suffering and depression. This is why I urge women to re-evaluate their priorities.

If any of these conservative therapies work, I jump up and down with elation and true joy for you. For those who have found anything but relief in these many treatment methods, this is an important issue. From family expectations to doctor's opinions, please remember that this is your body and your life.

I remember countless times when I felt intimidated by my physician whenever I would bring up the subject of hysterectomy. I was made to feel as if I weren't enough of a trouper, a fighter or a player. I finally realized that this was not a game I wanted to play, and that I wasn't helping anyone, least of all myself. My relationships suffered, my work suffered, and, most of all, my sense of self and self-esteem suffered. I felt as if I weren't as strong as I should be, and that I could not handle the situations I believed were supposed to be handled with ease.

——— ◊ ———

What I found is that *it was not my fault*.
There was and is nothing wrong with me.
It is the endometriosis, not me.
——— ◊ ———

Because there are varying degrees of the disease, it is hard to determine where you fall in the scale of severity. Your first laparoscopy can best be evaluated for future lesions and severity. If you have exhausted, as I did, all possibilities, this is another indication of what your future with the disease may bring. Not only did I exhaust the options, I did it three or four times. I don't want this to happen to you. This can wreak havoc on even the strongest of women.

——— ◊ ———

Don't feel ashamed, embarrassed or intimidated
if you are depleted.
——— ◊ ———

Know that you have options and information.

Each woman is her own powerhouse; and it is amazing what we can do as a whole. Contact support groups. The Endometriosis Research Center is an amazing group that is on the cutting edge of all options. I am a member, and I recommend it to everyone who has this disease. The Endometriosis Research Center provides a list of women you can contact for support, guidance or to lend a friendly ear. (For more information, see chapter 10)

SURGICAL TREATMENTS

When is surgery indicated? Many facets of a woman's life must be taken into account when considering surgery. Treatment is individualized. The first step can be an exploratory surgery called a laparoscopy. This can determine if you have the disease, and your doctor can excise existing lesions if they are present, but this is not a cure. There is no cure for endometriosis. This is just a maintenance method and is usually temporary. Subsequent laparoscopies can remove newer lesions but in turn may leave more scarring and tissue damage. Laparoscopies, which include a LUNA, can help reduce dysmenorrhea, but again, pain may not be reduced significantly enough for a woman to use that as her definitive surgery.

There are several techniques that can be performed during a laparoscopy, and it is up to you and your doctor to decide. In a laparoscopy, a tiny incision is made through the belly button and gas is blown into the abdomen so the surgeon can easily see the pelvic region. This is also to ensure that the surgeon does not puncture any of the surrounding organs.

While performing a laparoscopy, your surgeon may opt to do a hysteroscopy. Hysteroscopy is a method in which the surgeon can view the inner walls of the uterus. A long periscope is inserted for visualization. Other surgical tools can be inserted through the scope to cut or remove abnormal tissue. The hysterescope is inserted through the vagina and then through the cervical opening into the heart of the uterus.

Your surgeon may want to perform a presacral neurectomy. This is a surgical procedure in which the nerves at the back of the uterus are severed in an attempt to eliminate or reduce pain associated with endometriosis. After such a surgery, the tissue will be sent to pathology for biopsy. Views of the uterus will be developed, and marked abnormalities can be seen. The main discomfort that the surgery poses is from the gas pain. Within three to four days your body will naturally eliminate the gas. Your chest and shoulders may also be uncomfortable because of the trapped gas, but this will be alleviated in a few days.

HYSTERECTOMY

Hysterectomy, removal of the uterus, or a total hysterectomy and Salpingo-oopherectomy (removal of uterus, ovaries, tubes and cervix) are options for the woman who has exhausted all other possibilities or who determines she is at a place in her life where fertility is not an issue. This is a delicate situation.

I was 27 when I had my total hysterectomy. It was certainly not an age a woman would want to hand over her fertility. But I definitely had enough of surgeries and drug therapies that were useless.

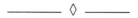

When I approached my physician for a hysterectomy, he sang the lawsuit blues, claiming he was under suit for performing a hysterectomy on a woman who then changed her mind.

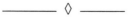

I can understand his hesitation but can't help but think that my pain and suffering would have been greatly reduced had I not had to jump around town for opinions. I went to another gynecologist.

Hesitance to perform definitive surgery varies among physicians. On my first visit to the female doctor who later assisted in performing my hysterectomy, she readily thought of hysterectomy as a very real approach. This is not to say she was careless or hasty. She examined my medical records and spoke with several other gynecologists who knew of my situation but had been reluctant to perform the surgery. She came through for me, acting as both a physician and liaison among all my other health-care providers.

She was clear about the seriousness of this decision but regarded my past as enough suffering. After 10 years, it was time for me to get my life back. I always wanted to have children but not at the expense of my health and life. I would be no good for them or anyone else. It was not even clear if I could carry a baby to term. As it turns out, I can have children, just not through this body. Adoption is a wonderful alternative for those who can't conceive, and I plan to do just that. The trade-off is so worth it for me. I look back to all the years I suffered and thank God for giving me the strength to make such a difficult decision.

Is hysterectomy a path for every woman to follow? Certainly not. For me, however, it was. I never regret my decision. I have a life that I had only before looked at through windows clouded by tears and pain. Although I understand that deep within me this disease may lurk, today I am free. For that I am grateful. For that, I am a woman forever living with endometriosis.

FREQUENTLY ASKED QUESTIONS ABOUT SURGERY

1. *What is a laparoscopy?*

    It's an exploratory surgical procedure to see what is happening inside your abdomen. A tiny incision is made in your navel, and your abdomen is filled with gas to better see all the abdominal organs. A slim laparascope is inserted, and the surgeon can see endometrial implants, cysts or any other foreign growth. These can be excised, cauterized or burned off with a laser.

2. *What is bowel prep?*

   It is used both to empty the bowel and colon and to kill bacteria in the area. Usually a liquid diet is prescribed a couple of days before surgery along with an enema or two the night before and morning of surgery. Your doctor may prescribe a liquid substance that will stimulate your bowels. Anti-infection drugs are also prescribed to kill bacteria in the area.

3. *What is the recovery time?*

   If all goes as planned with a laparoscopy, you will be out of the hospital by the end of the day. You should be up and around in a few days, capable of all but high-impact activities and intercourse. It may be a couple of weeks before these can be performed with comfort.

   With a hysterectomy, recovery time depends on the type of surgery. If it is vaginal, you should only be in the hospital a day or two. If it is abdominal, you may be in from three to six days. Recovery is slow, and you must not lift anything heavy, do any strenuous activities or have sex for at least four weeks.

4. *What is a LUNA?*

   A LUNA, or uterosacral nerve ablation, is a procedure in which the uterosacral ligaments are severed to relieve centralized pain. This procedure also relieves pain associated with dysmenorrhea. LUNA is not as effective in relieving pain associated with adhesions, endometriomas or pelvic endometriosis.

5. *What is a presacral neurectomy?*

   It is a surgical procedure in which the nerves at the back of the uterus are severed in an attempt to reduce or eliminate pain. This is most effective for centralized pain.

6. *When will I know if it "worked"?*

   Don't be dismayed if your first period after surgery is heavy and painful; it's common. Give it some time, a month or two, to notice any real relief. Time may vary, depending on the location and severity of the endometriosis.

~

~Chapter Three~

You & Your Doctor

How To Become Your Own Advocate While Retaining Your Dignity

You should approach your health provider with a sense of self and self-dignity. After all, you are a competent individual who is aware of her own body. You should be armed with knowledge of your particular concerns and feel comfortable to speak freely and easily with your provider.

To be your own advocate, you must overcome certain prevailing realities. As much as your physician would like to, she or he may not be current on all of the newest and most effective technologies and developments associated with your situation.

———— ◊ ————

Do your own research, and be able
to understand what your options are.

———— ◊ ————

Patient and physician must create a mutually effective relationship. As much as doctors can lead us to information and work with us, they cannot work entirely for us. Empower yourself by being an active participant in your health care. Your doctor will appreciate and respect you more.

———— ◊ ————

Use the physician as you would a friend, not a god.

———— ◊ ————

It used to be that I didn't feel good about the exchanges I had with my doctors. Then I found a gynecologist with whom I felt comfortable speaking regarding all issues relating to my disease, including sexual, psychological and emotional issues.

When speaking to your doctor, present your case as if you were writing an outline for a book. Write down your questions and concerns before your appointment and ferret out any related issues.

For example:

Question: What do I do about the pain?

Options:

1. OTC drugs
2. narcotic/prescriptions
3. relaxation

Knowing your options comes only out of doing your homework before meeting with your doctor.

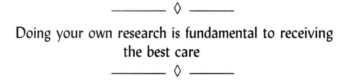

Doing your own research is fundamental to receiving the best care

To further improve your knowledge, take paper and pencil with you to write down the topics of discussion. You may also opt for a small tape recorder if you want to listen to what your doctor said in full detail later. Some women benefit from keeping all their appointments and research in one notebook. Keeping a diary also prompts questions you may want to pose to your doctor. Chapter Nine is devoted to helping you document your concerns and progress.

Questions to ask your doctor:

1. What are the benefits of doing this?
2. What are the risks?
3. What are my other options?

4. What should I do first?

5. What are the probable outcomes of each situation?

6. What is the probable outcome if I decide not to have this treatment?

The doctor will invariably ask what your pain is like and where it is. Be prepared.

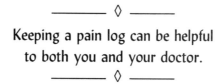

Keeping a pain log can be helpful
to both you and your doctor.

It is important to know when and where your pain is localized. This information can help determine which times of the month and where you are most sensitive.

Localizing your pain can also assist the doctor to determine if there is a cyst on your ovary or centralized pain from your uterus. There are medical explanations for each area. Again, do the legwork before seeing your doctor. Information is power.

GETTING MORE COMFORTABLE

Let your doctor know if you are uptight during an exam. Maybe your doctor hasn't noticed that you're clinging to the ceiling. My former gynecologist had "Where's Waldo" pictures on the ceiling, and it really helped.

But pain can't be ignored or averted with a cartoon character. During the exam, if I wasn't in the stirrups I surely would have knocked the doctor out with one fell swoop.

It's O.K. to ask your doctor to stop the exam. It's your body and your pain.

Here are ideas for your doctor that may help the exam be more tolerable for the both of you:

1. Pad stirrups with socks or oven mitts.

2. Put scenic or interesting posters on the ceiling.

3. Warm the instruments using friction or a lamp before use.

4. Have the procedure explained to you before and during the exam.

5. Use "comfortable" terminology. For example, "Let your legs fall apart," instead of "Spread your legs."

QUESTIONS ABOUT SURGERY

If you are scheduled for a laparoscopy, be informed about what is going to be done and what possible findings will render what treatment. Ask about anesthesia and the post-operative pain. You will speak with the anesthesiologist before your surgery, and she or he will answer your questions. Again, write them down beforehand so you feel confident you have covered all of your concerns.

After surgery, discuss in detail with the doctor the findings and the action taken. The doctor will usually not be present in the recovery room, so it is important to seek answers to your questions as soon as possible.

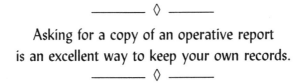

Asking for a copy of an operative report
is an excellent way to keep your own records.

Have your doctor discuss the report with you to ensure you understand the jargon. After you have your answers, you can jointly discuss realistic treatments.

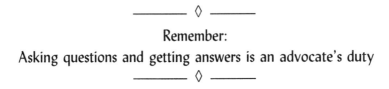

Remember:
Asking questions and getting answers is an advocate's duty

HELP, I CAN'T STAND MY DOCTOR!

Here are seven signs that you may need to change doctors:

1. You can't talk freely and easily with your doctor about your health without embarrassment or fear of reprisal.

2. You must communicate primarily through the staff and not the doctor.

3. The office staff is rude, incompetent or unhelpful.

4. Your doctor is not including you in discussions regarding your health.

5. Your doctor is not able to see you regularly.

6. You can't reach your doctor easily, and she or he does not respond to you within a reasonable time.

7. Your doctor is not listening to you.

If you are having trouble with your current physician or the medical staff, make a change.

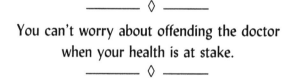

**You can't worry about offending the doctor
when your health is at stake.**

Ask the receptionist to transfer your medical records to your new doctor. This is your body and your choice.

I remember when I was having trouble with my former gynecologist. He was an opinionated individual who got frustrated easily and we were always sparring. He would write belittling notes in my medical records. I discovered this only after I requested a copy of my records. You can get a copy of your medical records whenever you like. These are your records, and you have the right to know what is in them

I called my former doctor once while experiencing pain. I told him I was at home working on my laptop but was in too much pain to go to the office to work. In my medical records he wrote: "She was sitting by the pool working on her laptop and *claims* she wants a hysterectomy and *claims* that the pain medication was not working." It read as if I were a child, feigning sickness to avoid a math quiz.

Whenever I ended up in the Emergency Room with unrelenting pain, he would blow in like a tornado, expressing his frustration and irritation by his hurried behavior and condescending tone. Many of the ER staff felt the same way I did about him, although their empathy didn't solve my problem.

The worst part was, I was afraid to see him. I would call only after experiencing tremendous, prolonged pain and distress. The thought of having to go to him for help about made me crawl out of my skin. Although he was a "book smart" physician, his bedside manner was non-existent. Because of this, my regard for his abilities as a doctor plummeted. I wanted both competence and compassion, as many women do, and I am glad I continued my search until I found a doctor who provided both.

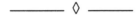

There is no perfect relationship between a patient and doctor, but you should feel you are being heard and understood.

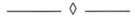

The frustrations you experience may go far beyond your primary provider. On several occasions I had to go to the ER with unmanageable pain and/or bleeding. Specifically, after a minor procedure, I had to go to the ER continuously because I could not urinate. Because I had been there so frequently, the staff knew my plight. But some were rude and negligent. I would hear them whisper that I was just in for a medicine fix and that I wasn't really in much pain.

After three weeks with a foley catheter, I was chastised by both my doctor and some of the ER staff for being unable to insert it myself. When your pain level is high you don't want to stick a tube up your urethra. Also, I wanted to know *why* I needed the catheter and could not urinate on my own. I wanted to find a solution, not maintain the problem.

Some members of the ER staff were openly annoyed by me. Once, when my catheter was leaking, the ER receptionist handed me a new one and said, "Here you go, the bathroom is over there." I was crying with pain and frightened that I needed a catheter. How could I put it in myself? I had just been there the night before, and the same staff knew I was not able to do that. My mother was a witness to this treatment. She helped me hold my ground and ask that I get help from a nurse. The receptionist said there would be a three-hour wait although it was after 2:00 AM and the waiting room was empty.

———— ◊ ————

If it happened to me, it can happen to you.

———— ◊ ————

Don't accept it. My only regret is that I neglected to get the names of those involved so I could write a letter to Patient Affairs.

If you ever have such an experience, get in touch with the facility's ombudsman who serves as a liaison between patients and doctors. This person will take down your complaint and anonymously bring it to the attention of the party named. You can follow up to see if any disciplinary action took place.

That evening in the ER deeply affected me and my treatment. When I experienced unmanageable pain or trouble with either the catheter or abnormal bleeding, I was too scared to return to the ER. I was embarrassed, ashamed and emotionally weak. I could not tolerate any more abuse. This is when I began to cry all the time, feeling so lost and afraid. If the health-care professionals were not there to help me, I asked myself, "What do I do?" Was I really crazy and as much of a nuisance as they thought? I have heard two physicians speak derogatorily about me when they didn't know I was listening. Great, there I was with my feet in stirrups, an IV in me, tears streaming down my face, shaking with anxiety over the prospect of what I had heard.

———— ◊ ————

As I grew stronger as a woman,
I realized that I was not paranoid and that
this was their problem, not mine.

———— ◊ ————

Without the continual support of my therapist, the strength of my mother and my faith in God, I would never have been able to endure the most unbearable of times.

———— ◊ ————

I vowed never to let a doctor or staff make me feel small
or insignificant again.

———— ◊ ————

If I have to, I will go to his face with a bull horn and firmly state what I am feeling. I will not pose it as a question or allow him the ability to dismiss me without being heard. We have to unite on this. Say it loud and clear and *make* them listen.

I have also had rewarding experiences with primary doctors and ER doctors and nurses. I wish to thank all of you (you know who you are). Thank you for adding to my sense of self instead of stunting it. Thank you for your smiles and your empathy and, most of all, your expertise.

Receiving quality health care is fundamental, and society should do everything it can to provide this. As much as I encourage you who feel abused by the profession to write a complaint letter, I equally and strongly suggest that we acknowledge those who did their best. So often people document only their bad experiences and just accept the good ones. I have written letters of thanks to both my physicians and the HMO they work for.

———— ◊ ————

Exemplary physicians and nurses should be acknowledged for
their dedication and regard.

———— ◊ ————

STRENGTH IN NUMBERS

The experiences I have had dealing with the disease for
10 years are mine only. I do not pretend to predict what
may happen or influence any woman to follow my path. I
just want the hand of opportunity to be there when a
woman feels she needs one. I speak from years of
heartache and turmoil. I speak in hope that I may be able
to help even one woman decide what is best for her. What
one woman alone cannot endure, collectively we can
achieve. For too long women have not been able to speak
freely and openly about their experiences with the disease.
I urge all women with the disease to reach out to others
for support and affirmation. There is a list of resources for
you in ChapterTen.

TIPS FOR HANDLING YOURSELF IN THE EMERGENCY ROOM

You're scared, in pain, bleeding or having some kind
of frightening and discerning symptom. It's after hours
and you have to go to the emergency room. Here are some
tips:

1. Speak up! If you are in agonizing pain or are bleeding
   heavily go to the front of the line and firmly state that
   you are in a state of distress. Relay the issue at hand
   succinctly and articulate well.

2. Have your insurance or identification card out.

3. Have the name of your gynecologist and/or primary
   physician.

4. Every fifteen minutes check with the receptionist; do
   not wait more than thirty minutes before stating the
   urgency of your being seen.

5. Once in a room, clearly explain your problem. If you are in pain, the doctor may ask what you would like them to do. *Do not feel intimidated*! Say that you need pain relief.

6. Be firm, yet assertive. Make certain your needs are met within an adequate amount of time. If the ER is busy, have a nurse make you as comfortable as possible until the doctor can see you.

7. Give the ER doctor as much information as you can about your health history, including medications. This will expedite your treatment.

8. Be honest. There is no shame in unmanageable pain.

9. Retain all records and see your regular doctor ASAP.

~

~Chapter Four~

Documenting Your Pain & Treatment

Sometimes your situation seems indescribable, yet describing it is usually the first step in getting help. I use two techniques, a pain scale and a journal.

The pain scale was given to me by a fellow endometriosis sufferer, and it's been invaluable. It really helps me put my life in perspective and helps me communicate my pain to doctors and nurses.

Being your own advocate means knowing your body and how it works. A pain scale can greatly assist your doctor in comprehending and treating your level of agony. It also helps to let the doctor know where the pain is, which is helpful because pains in different areas of the abdomen indicate different probable causes. If you are in a hospital for pain management or recovering from a surgery, it is likely that the nurses will periodically ask you about your pain level. Being familiar with this scale is an effective way for you to communicate to those treating your pain.

MANKOSKI PAIN SCALE

0 = Pain-free.

1 = Very minor annoyance.

2 = Minor annoyance.

3 = Annoying enough to be distracting; need mild painkillers.

4 = Distracting; mild painkillers remove pain for three to four hours.

5 = Can't be ignored for more than 30 minutes; need mild painkillers.

6 = Can't be ignored at all; stronger painkillers needed.

7 = Difficulty concentrating, sleeping; stronger painkillers ineffective.

8 = Physical activity severely limited; nausea and dizziness.

9 = Unable to speak; crying out and moaning; near delirium.

10 = Unconscious.

I also keep a daily pain journal that helps me understand when the pain is at its worst. This substantiates to me that I am suffering.

It is a good idea to keep a journal of your trials with endometriosis. Begin with your first signs of pain or diagnosis, and document each doctors' appointment, surgery (and operative report), medical treatment and assessment. You may also want to include some personal feelings.

This is not only cathartic, but also allows you to have complete documentation of your treatment path. If you suffer with endometriosis for 10 years, as I did, you will find it helpful to have your earliest treatments, suggestions and thoughts written down. This will help you make decisions based on your health history, and it can be of enormous help to both you and your physician.

Samples of my journal are included in Chapter 9.

CASE HISTORY

I received thousands of letters and e-mail from women around the world, and a few were kind enough to write down the course of their trials and tribulations in dealing with endometrosis. Here is an amazingly detailed account of one woman's experience:

TIMELINE

5/7/88   Approximate date of pregnancy.

6/1/88   Family doctor confirmed pregnancy, referred to OB-GYN.

7/19/88   Pap Smear. Yeast infection. Mild to moderate inflammation.

2/9/89   Went to OB-GYN. Complained of pain in lower right abdomen.

3/21/89   Pap smear. Mild to moderate inflammation.

10/9/89   Complained to doctor of dyspareunia and recurrent intermittent vaginal burning.

10/31/89   Bad yeast infection.

3/22/90   Check-up; everything fine.

4/12/91   Pap smear. Severe inflammation, vaginitus (never told by doctor).

11/8/91   Tubal ligation.

12/6/91   Check-up after tubal ligation; pain in my lower right quadrant; nausea and tenderness. Doctor said possible abdominal wall strain or intestinal discomfort.

8/18/92   Pain in lower right quadrant usually at period time.

Doctor assessment: There is some tenderness in the right side mid-abdomen up toward the liver. Some tenderness still present with the rectus muscles under tension. Abdominal pain possibly from abdominal wall strain. Irritable colon pain. She may have some referred pain in in the area at the menstrual time. *PLAN*: Return in one year for next check up or sooner if indicated or if pain worsens we will consider laparoscopies.

8/20/92   Pap smear. Moderate inflammation.

10/5/92   Missed September period. Right lower quadrant pain. Spotting, breast tenderness. PMS symptoms only 12 times worse.

9/16/93   Pap smear. Severe inflammation.

2/23/93   Right lower quadrant pain all the time. Vaginal odor that worsens at period time.

3/11/93   Right lower quadrant pain. Mother has a history of colon problems. Odor and discharge.

Doctor assessment: Abdomen tender, especially in the descending colon. Severe chronic cervictitis. Blood in stool, referred to GI.

3/25/93   Cyrosurgery done.

3/31/93   Colonoscopy done. Diagnosed with spastic colon.

3/1/94   Went on vacation in Houston/ Galveston and got sick. I went to the Texas Medical Center in Galveston and they diagnosed me with pelvic inflammatory disease. (I did not even know what that was). I was so embarrassed when I got home and read it was a sexually transmitted disease. I have only one sex partner, my husband.

3/11/94   Returned home and saw my doctor. Had some dyspareunia, seen in ER in Galveston for severe right lower quadrant pain, shortness of breath and dizziness.

Doctor assessment: Abdomen soft. She does have some tenderness in the lower quadrant. Questionable tenderness in the abdominal wall. Acute abdominal pain, probably intestinal colic, doubt pelvic infection. Periods are becoming heavier and more painful. Placed on Anaprox for abdominal discomfort.

3/11/94   Pap smear. Mild inflammation.

10/6/94   Increasing dyspareunia to the point of painful intercourse. Also has had severe dysmenorrhea.

Doctor assessment: Some tenderness in the cul-de-sac. Progressive dysmenorrhea and dyspareunia. Rule out endometriosis. The patient will keep a diary to evaluate where pain is coming from and to help make a diagnosis and correct the measures. In reviewing her menstrual chart, she appears to be ovulatory, but her periods are heavy. She also may consider with the laparoscopy a diagnostic hysteroscopy to be sure there are no polyps or other causes of her heavy bleeding.

10/12/94   Pap smear. Moderate inflammation.

10/14/94   *Pre-operative diagnosis*: Severe dysmenorrhea. Rule out endometriosis.

Post-operative diagnosis: Endometriosis involving left uterosacral ligament and cul-de-sac.

Operation: Diagnostic and operative laparoscopy with cauterization of endometrial implants.

Procedure: There was a corpus lutem on the right ovary. Left ovary was normal. Exam of cul-de-sac, however, revealed endometriosis involving the cul-de-sac and the left uterosacral ligament. Most of them were in the form of small dirt spots and "powder burns." The liver and gallbladder appeared to be normal. The appendix was never seen. Using the bipolar forceps the endometriotic lesions were very carefully cauterized until totally ablated.

11/11/94   Return for post-op exam. Last period after surgery was heaviest of all. Continue to keep track of these.

4/20/95   Continue to have severe dysmenorrhea. Pain in the right lower quadrant and pain with intercourse.

Doctor assessment: I am suspicious that this could possibly be abdominal wall pain. The central pain, however, I believe is probably secondary to her endometriosis. She did have relief for a couple of months but the discomfort has returned. Abdominal pain, possibly abdominal wall. Severe dysmenorrhea probably secondary to endometriosis. Will consider Lupron for a few months Has had tubal sterilization, will consider definitive management with hysterectomy probably trying to preserve the ovaries at this time.

Note: The doctor told me on numerous occasions that the pain was being caused by stress or that it was all in my head. I had to beg him to do the laparoscopy in 1994. In April 1995, when I told him the endometriosis was back, he told me it did not come back and that it was all in my head. See above doctor assessment.

3/25/96   Saw new doctor. Gave options of continual laparoscopies, Depo-Provera, Lupron and hysterectomy.

4/19/96   Took injection of Depo-Provera. Continual bleeding until 6/7/96.

6/5/96   Declined Lupron injection because of the expense and no long-term cure. Scheduled hysterectomy.

6/7/96   Ultrasound; fine.

6/18/96   Hysterectomy. Became anemic, had two units of blood transfused from family members. Had hematoma on bladder due to internal bleeding. Depo-Provera injection given after surgery.

Stayed in hospital for five days. Discharged 6/23/96.

6/25/96   Went to doctor with fever of 101.5, racing pulse, nausea. Ultrasound: Gallbladder wall had increased to double its normal thickness and there were several localized areas that are nonshadowing and probably due to areas of "sludge." There is a fluid collection in the right lower pelvic area and two rounded areas with irregular margination in the pelvic area that could be due to hematoma and abscess. A pelvic CT scan was recommended to differentiate pelvic abscess that could be drained at this time. Admitted back to hospital for three days.

7/1/96   Check up. Vaginal cuff healing well.

7/15/96   Ultrasound. Post-op hematoma or abscess is considered most likely. Today mass measures 3.6 x 2.4 x 4 cm.

7/17/96   Feel much better, but continued discomfort voiding and pressure over hematoma. Low-grade urinary infection.

8/7/96   Difficult to even feel hematoma. Started Ogen 1.25 mg. daily.

9/4/96   Estrogen is low. Injection given and increase to 2.50 Ogen daily.

9/24/96   Pain in bladder. Urine test negative for infection.

9/26/96   Ultrasound. Pelvic mass measures 4 x 3 x 2.4 cm. Marked interval decrease in the probable postoperative hematoma just above the vaginal cuff. There was also some scarring noted in the left lower quadrant. There was dense area of endometriosis and scar tissue from the rectum to the back portion to the top of the vagina. The suction irrigation probe was used to dissect the colon away from the top of the vagina as safely as possible. There was a small remaining area, not necessary to further proceed with carbon dioxide laser due to the close proximity to the colon. Recommended to undergo three to six months of Lupron therapy.

11/20/96 Urine test done for infection, negative. Referred to urologist.

11/22/96 Saw urologist and had a cytoscopy that revealed trigonitus on the bladder floor. It was very red and infected. Pus and blood in urine. On antibiotics until 1/10/97.

11/27/96 Received first Lupron injection and was informed that the endometriosis was worse. It was now up on my intestines and OB-GYN could not get it all for fear of burning a hole in intestines.

12/11/96 Severe pain from endometriosis. Ultrasound performed showed everything to be normal. The doctor indicated that I was having a reaction to the Lupron injection that was responsible for the flare-up.

12/23/96 Lupron injection.

1/21/97 Lupron injection.

1/24/97 Called doctor with more pain and went in for a blood test on my liver. Tests came back fine.

1/28/97 Saw doctor and continued to have pain in my side around my liver area and lower back. Have continued off and on pain medications and anti-inflammatory medications that don't seem to work. My doctor said she had checked with manufacturer and was told that after the third, if no improvements are made, then there is no reason to continue taking the shots. She suggested I see a counselor to deal with my problems, pain, depression etc.

1/29/97   Made an appointment with a counselor. Contacted an association and was told that I don't need a counselor if I have a supportive family. I was put in contact with a reproductive endocrinologist at the Oklahoma University Health Science. I have an appointment 2/4/97.

What an ordeal! Can you relate to any of the frustrations and repeated tests and drugs prescribed? I sure can! By the way, this woman is 29. She is a hero in my eyes and has endured so much pain with grace and dignity. She has also had strength enough to share her story with me so I could share it with all of you.

I welcome your letters, documents and thoughts. Please write me at the address shown in the resources or e-mail me at Bucalu@aol.com. Your insights will help other women who have endometriosis as well as their families.

~

CHAPTER FIVE

PREPARING FOR SETBACKS

The debilitating effects of endometriosis extend far beyond the women with the disease. The disease effects every aspect of a woman's life: her mental state, finances and relationships. When I say relationships, I include husbands, boyfriends, lovers, children, employer-employee and friends. When a woman is in chronic pain, it depletes her mental and physical strength and her ability to give herself to loved ones. Formerly enjoyable sex becomes a feared nightmare, and keeping up with kids is a frustrating impossibility. Dates with friends are canceled because "she's not up to it," and everyone begins to feel neglected.

Recognize that stress on relationships is a reality and that the most important action you can take is to care for yourself. Talk about your frustrations with your significant other and friends.

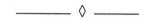

Keep the lines of communication open and reassure them that this is no one's fault; not yours, not theirs.

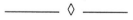

Explain your sense of futility at not being able to meet the needs of others, nor your own. After all, we would like nothing more than to go back to enjoying sex and romping with the little ones. Sometimes we can't, and that, too, is OK.

Please be good to yourself and try not to place any more guilt on your shoulders. I have received letters from husbands who simply don't know what to do. They wish they could take away the pain their loved one suffers because when we hurt, they hurt (this is addressed in Chapter 7).

You may have small children who cannot understand why Mommy is sick. They are frightened and uncertain.

——— ◊ ———

Reassure them that they are not the reason you are ill.

——— ◊ ———

Compare it to when they have a tummy ache and explain to them that you need some quiet time. Getting some peace can be especially difficult if you are a single mother. Schedule quiet time for all of you to draw, listen to music or read. Finances may be tight, but if you can swing it, have a baby-sitter come in a few times a week to give you a break. Also, look for resources in your community. Support groups offer alternatives and suggestions for both you and your loved ones. If we stick together, we can work it out.

LOST WAGES

This is a sensitive subject, but it needs to be addressed. There are so many intricate details involved when applying for either disability or unemployment. When you submit your claim you will be drilled on the reason you are not working. Your physician's documentation may also affect your claim.

I was not employed when I had my hysterectomy. I had to stop working before surgery because I was in debilitating pain most of the time and my work was affected. My stamina and concentration were totally diffused, and I found myself struggling just to hold on until 5 p.m., when I would go home and climb directly into bed with my dog, Artie. When I applied for disability after my hysterectomy, my claim was rendered ineligible because I had left the labor force five months earlier. I was disappointed, because I felt I had a right to what I would have made during the six weeks of my recovery.

——— ◊ ———

**I had no idea that I should have had a doctor document all
the months I spent in pain.**

——— ◊ ———

Having the doctor do this after the fact is usually ineffective but worth a try.

If you are denied disability, you can appeal through writing to the State Disability Office in your area, which I encourage you to do. I was not seeking anything more than what I would have made during my recovery period, but I asked too late, and I don't want you to make the same mistake.

——— ◊ ———

**I do not agree with "cheating the system" and urge anyone
applying for disability to remain above reproach.**

——— ◊ ———

As much as I think my refusal was unfair, I understand the reasoning. The only real mistake was my not looking into it sooner. Had I had documentation of my inability to work, I would have received benefits. So speak up! You deserve it! People with injuries that prevent them from working are granted disability every day, including women suffering from endometriosis or recovering from a hysterectomy.

Not being able to make ends meet is scary. I was lucky to have help from my parents, but many women don't have that luxury. Some sufferers have children whose basic needs seem endless. The long-term effects on a family can be devastating. Those relying on dual incomes are suddenly faced with financial insecurity or debt. In addition to time off work, the medical treatments cost a significant sum. If I did not have insurance through a previous job, I am sure I would still be suffering. Why? Because I could not have afforded the treatment necessary for my optimal health.

Each day I hear from women who cannot receive quality care because their insurance will not cover the expensive hormonal treatments or surgical procedures. This infuriates me. I heard from a woman who had been diagnosed with probable endometriosis. (The doctor she had seen earlier that year had felt what he thought to be nodules upon physical examination). When she attempted to get insurance to cover treatment, she could not find an affordable carrier that would accept pre-existing conditions. This is not uncommon.

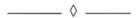

Women need to really research their insurance (or lack thereof) and make an educated decision based on their needs

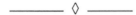

You can urge your employer to carry another policy or appeal your case to the board of the HMO or Independent Health organization. I have done it, and it works. Remember to stay strong and focused. You can do it!

DEPRESSION

For reasons both physiological and psychological, depression can be a very real part of endometriosis. Those of you who feel alone in this, don't! You are among a great many who suffer silently, as I did for years. Whether you are embarrassed or angry with yourself for not being able to "snap out of it," don't despair. You are normal! There are many ways you can help your depression. I speak from experience.

The definition of depression is "a state of despondency characterized by feelings of inadequacy, lowered activity and pessimism about the future, an extreme state of unresponsiveness to stimuli, together with self-depreciation, delusions of inadequacy and hopelessness." Sadly, this definition implies a defect of character or weakness because you are suffering. Nothing is further from the truth.

There are many biochemical reasons why your depression exists. Women on hormonal therapies such as Danazol, Synarel or Lupron experience a state of menopause in which their levels of naturally occurring hormones are dramatically diminished. Nueroendocrine studies have shown correlation between depression and hormone deficiencies.

In surgery, nerves are cut, and this destroys endocrine organs that produce hormones, thus eliciting fewer hormones and creating a biological state of depression. The deficiency of tryptophan and beta endorphins plays a large role in depression. For women on hormonal therapy in which estrogen levels are reduced, tryptophan is reduced as well. Patients treated with antidepressants that include tryptophan have shown an increase in brain endorphin levels. Naturally produced brain endorphins are stifled with hormonal therapies, which can result in depression.

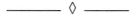

When I put a message up on my Web site, many women wrote of their experiences with depression.

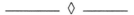

Several of the women I spoke with are held captive by feelings of futility and despair because they have exhausted so many options and are still experiencing pain and discomfort. I was reminded of myself and how depressed I became as a direct result of this disease and of my inability to stop the pain. When I was in the hospital, my temperature rose periodically to 100 degrees. The doctor on rounds said that pain can elevate temperature. I was surprised that the mere presence of pain can have such a dramatic effect on one's internal thermostat. It really put it in perspective how much the body is affected by pain. I could better understand how a consistently high pain level could physiologically cause depression.

Equally important are external factors that can cause depression, as addressed in the beginning of this chapter: finances, relationships, stress, among others.

If you consistently feel sad or despondent, seek help. Choose a therapist who specializes in chronic pain or women's issues. Your knowledgeable therapist will not only reassure you that you are normal, but also explain that there may be a medical solution to your depression. Many factors play a role in feeling low, including, but not limited to: nutrition; hormones; exercise or lack thereof; lack of family or spousal support; and lack of faith in your health provider. All of these need to be taken into account when seeking help and finding a solution. Simple changes in diet or exercise may dramatically help fade depression.

In conjunction with medical therapy, I found that talking to other women who had the same disease helped me. That is why I encourage every woman with endometriosis to join an association or support group. You will never be alone again. It helped a great deal to hear about other women's experiences and what they learned from them.

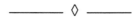

After hearing many other "respectable" women share their stories, my self-hatred stopped.

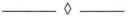

It is not your fault that you have endometriosis and all of the baffling and painful symptoms that accompany it.

After my devastating experience in the ER, I became isolated. I ended a four-year relationship that was greatly affected by my disease. The negativity and futility of my situation spread like a virus through my relationships not only with him, but also my friends, my work and my family. I became depressed and began to rely on my medications to take me from the misery and pain. I thought prescription medicine was the only "relationship" I could count on. At the time, it seemed that no one understood what I was enduring on a daily basis. To be honest, few did.

Isolation can be a very real contributor to depression. Those of us who have had or do have debilitating pain understand that it is not as simple as wanting to participate in our own lives. It is that we cannot do so. When we are unable to contribute financially, take the kids for a walk to the park, get an important project finished or make love with our partner, we suffer. But don't give up. Most depression is treatable.

The good news is depression can be treated successfully through lifestyle changes, psycho-therapy and antidepressants. A woman can take antidepressants while she is undergoing hormonal therapy. Any time you take a drug, there are alterations in your environment. You and your doctor can decide the best method of therapy for you.

I am not sure what is worse, crying for help and not being heard or calling for help and having the person who hears you diminish or trivialize your problem. This can trigger emotions that are the ingredients for full-blown depression.

I cannot stress this enough: It is always a good idea for a woman to have someone to talk with about her feelings, a friend, physician or therapist. Stepping out of yourself and sharing with others greatly reduces stress and negativity. You are not the only one.

~

~Chapter Six~

Life After A Hysterectomy

So the uterus and whatever else are history. The pain level is tolerable and, once again, the white slacks can come out of the closet. Now what? Brace yourself. Let me begin by saying that a hysterectomy is not a cure-all. Endometriosis can attack your bladder, rectum, colon, bowels and abdominal wall. In rare cases it has been found on the lung or appendix (if the appendix has not been removed during the hysterectomy). I had stubborn growths appear on my rectum four months after surgery.

However, and this is a big however, having the hysterectomy gave me my life back. I knew the pros and cons before going into surgery, and the pros smashed the cons to pieces! Having a hysterectomy was one of the most determined decisions I have ever made. I had been compromising my quality of life for far too long. Life consists of compromises. I made an educated and informed compromise.

There are several degrees of endometriois and several types of what people generalize as a "hysterectomy." Here are a few of the more common ones. Remember, this is a decision for you and your surgeon to discuss.

1. Myomectomy: Removes only the diseased portion of the uterus and surrounding areas.

2. Subtotal hysterectomy: Done vaginally, the cervix remains intact.

3. Total hysterectomy: Removes uterus and cervix leaving ovaries and tubes intact.

4. Total hysterectomy including tubes and ovaries (otherwise referred to as a hysterectomy with bilateral salpingo-oopherectomy): total removal of the uterus, both ovaries, tubes and cervix.

5. Radical hysterectomy: This procedure is most commonly used when cancer is present in reproductive organs. A large "margin" of the vagina is removed to lower the risk of recurrent cancer.

There are many considerations to be made when choosing the "right" surgery for you. It is contingent upon the severity and location of the endometriosis as well as your reproductive goals. Depending on which surgery you choose, there are different methods of removal. Hysterectomy and myomectomy can be done through the vagina using a laparascope, while more complete surgeries require either a horizontal or vertical incision in the abdomen.

———— ◊ ————

Preparation is vital not only to your physical health but also to your psyche.

———— ◊ ————

Find a surgeon with whom you feel comfortable, someone who can answer your questions and explain realistic goals of the surgery as well as any risks. Remember, this is a serious surgery, and you deserve the best. Preparing your body, mind and soul are imperative for a safe procedure and speedy recovery.

In Chapter Three, we looked at questions that you may wish to ask your doctor. Here are some examples of questions directly related to your surgery:

1. How long will the procedure take?

2. How long will I be hospitalized?

3. What are the risks during and after surgery?

4. What kind of anesthesia will be used and what are the risks?

5. What about diet and exercise before and after surgery?

6. What should I do to place my body is optimal health for surgery?

7. What pre-op meds do I need and what post-op meds do I need? Should I get them now to avoid hassle after surgery?

8. Will I or my family donate blood beforehand? When, where and how much should I donate?

9. Will I have a catheter? What kind?

10. Will I have an I.V.? What will be given to me intravenously?

11. When can I resume work, driving, bathing, sports, sex?

12. How many times have you done this? (If he says you're the guinea pig, RUN!!)

13. What types of hormonal treatments will I be placed on afterward and what purpose do they serve?

14. Anything else I should know?

Having these questions answered before surgery will calm and reassure you.

Finding a peaceful state of mind will enhance not only your pre-operative disposition but also your post-op. I found great strength and serenity through spiritual practices such as meditation and relying on a higher power to guide me. Whether you're agnostic, atheist or a firm believer, in times of crisis and confusion, thinking of a source other than yourself can help you achieve a serene state.

Along with my belief in God, I imagined my dog, Artie, and how much happiness he gave me, how calm, safe and serene I felt with him by my side.

CARING FOR YOURSELF

You made it through surgery, yet post-operatively you are in pain and hating each and every nurse who says it's time to get out of bed and stretch your legs. Uh! No way, not me! Although it seems impossible at the time, you can take that first step. And your second and third and so on. Eventually you'll be cruising the halls with your I.V. in tow, very proud of your accomplishments. And let me tell you, what an accomplishment it is! But take it easy.

——— ◊ ———

Your body has undergone a trauma, and it is up to you to nurse yourself back to health.

——— ◊ ———

You can do it. It may hurt tremendously the first day or so, but keep thinking about the months and years of debilitating pain you had with endometriosis. You are a strong and courageous woman who has had more than her fair share of the pits, and now you're on your way to the cherries, baby!

I WANTED THIS FOR SO LONG, SO WHY AM I SO SAD?

Give yourself a break! Remember, your body and mind need time to heal. Depending on the type of incision you had, recovery and the length of hospitalization may vary from three to ten days. Recovery from hysterectomy is a time-consuming process. Understanding this process as well as preparing for it before surgery will ease your post-operative stress, physiologically and psychologically.

About a week after my surgery it seemed all I could do was cry. I hurt physically, though the pain seemed to emanate from my heart, my soul. Although I did not know it then, depression after hysterectomy is normal. It can be brought on by many factors, including hormonal levels, incapacitation and the finality of the circumstances. For me, the realities of the situation were difficult. Did I want to have a total hysterectomy at 27? No, I elected to because I knew I could not compromise my quality of life any longer. The endometriosis left me bruised and battered, and my body and mind were overwhelmed.

I wanted children. The reality was such that I would never be able to bear them. It did not matter that I had come to terms with this consequence long before my hysterectomy, I was melancholy for all the "could be's" and "never will's."

Most women who lose the ability to conceive and reproduce experience an innate sense of loss.

——— ◊ ———

Grieving is a natural part of healing.

——— ◊ ———

All the pre-op appointments and preparations are over, and a complete emotional upheaval is taking place inside you. It is not only OK to cry and let your feelings go, it is also normal and enormously therapeutic. Don't deny yourself this aspect of the post-operative recovery process. Let your body guide you.

Ask your doctor to check your hormonal levels. The right amount of hormones can do wonders in balancing your perspective. As always, alert your physician to any abnormal bleeding from the vagina or incision area, or any other aspect of the recovery process that is unclear to you.

——— ◊ ———

If you need reassurance about anything, consult your physician. This is your right.

——— ◊ ———

WHY DO I STILL HAVE PAIN AFTER MY HYSTERECTOMY?

This seems to be the million-dollar question, and I wish I could give you a straight answer. If a total hysterectomy is performed with removal of all endometrial implants, why does the pelvic pain persist? Aside from pain because of undiscovered disease, adhesions or scar tissue from past surgeries can cause as much pain as the endometrial implants themselves. Where does that leave those of us who have had or who are thinking about having a hysterectomy to treat endometriosis?

That post-hysterectomy women experience pain clearly exposes the fallacy that hysterectomy "cures" endometriosis. However, hysterectomy can bring about great relief of symptoms, such as those awful periods and that unpredictable and heavy bleeding. Remember that every woman is different, and some experience nothing at all while others still suffer. It comes down to a personal choice, because there are so many differing opinions about this controversial topic. Again, do your homework and make an educated decision based on the facts.

THERE *IS* GREAT SEX AFTER SURGERY

I remember nights when I would be writhing in pain and my now-former boyfriend would hint about sex. You know what I am talking about. I remember countless days and nights when my sense of myself as a sexual being was buried because I could not enjoy foreplay or intercourse. I writhed at the thought of a foreign part inside my abdomen. By this time, I associated touching with the pain I experienced with exams and could not bear being touched unless absolutely necessary.

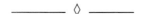

If a friend told me that one day I would actually desire sex,
I would have thought her delusional.
I am happy to report that it's indeed a fact!

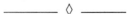

A hysterectomy may change your life, but it doesn't have to hinder it. It was a few months after the hysterectomy before I had intercourse, and the first few times were a little painful. As the body produces less estrogen, the walls of the vagina become drier and less elastic. Sex may be uncomfortable because of lack of moisture, but these physical—not-in-your-head—changes can be rectified with vaginal creams and lubricants. Your doctor may want to check your estrogen levels to make sure they are at therapeutic levels.

Gradually the surgical pain decreased, and I began to experience sex as a whole new phenomenon. Gone were the days of wide-eyed terror and anticipation mixed with dread. I was free! It was a truly liberating experience. I began to explore my sensuality.

———— ◊ ————

I felt feminine in every sense of the word.

———— ◊ ————

This was one side of me that had been dormant for so long I thought it had all but disappeared. I am not saying sexuality is the most important aspect of being a woman, because it is not. It can, however, have great negative impact on a woman's self-esteem and sense of well-being if she is unable to express herself, especially sexually. The endometriosis became a barrier between the rest of the world and me. Sex was just one aspect of my isolation.

If you are having difficulty making love, please be good to yourself. You do not deserve to feel, or be made to feel, inadequate. This is not a situation you have control over. Your body is in major chaos, and you desperately need to conserve all your positive energy so you can heal.

———— ◊ ————

Sex will be troublesome as long as you have endometriosis.

———— ◊ ————

I wish there were a magical remedy I could give each woman, but there isn't. For me, it took a complete hysterectomy. I hope it takes less radical surgery for others.

Should you decide to have a hysterectomy, know that you will get better and you will be able to resume innumerable activities once impossible to perform. Sex with my husband is now a regular part of my life. More important, I don't end up huddled in the fetal position, clutching my heating pad or wiping the tears that would inevitably be streaming down my face.

HORMONE REPLACEMENT THERAPY (HRT)

The issue of hormone replacement therapy is extremely controversial. Still, most of us have experienced hormonal therapy to some extent. Lupron, Danazol, Synarel and Depo-Provera, as well as many others, are often prescribed to combat endometriosis. All these drugs are intricately involved with our hormonal structure. In other words, they make us crazy! Seriously, the right balance of hormones post-hysterectomy is essential for synchronizing both our bodies and minds

Hormone replacement therapy is a means of "replacing" estrogen to its premenopausal level in your body. It is aimed at making your transition into menopause better with the fewest number of side effects. Menopause occurs when menstruation ceases naturally or when a surgical procedure, such as a hysterectomy, removes the ovaries along with the uterus. This is known as "surgical menopause." The average age of women who experience the first signs of natural menopause is 51. However, natural menopause can occur from the late 20s to the mid-50s.

Three kinds of hormones constitute HRT: estrogen, progesterone and testosterone. Estrogen is fundamental for maintaining overall health, including bone density, low cholesterol, healthy skin, vaginal moisture and many other functions. Progesterone can reduce the incidence of breast cancer and can elevate your endorphins (those naturally occurring "happy hormones"). Testosterone may or may not be necessary in your HRT but can help increase your sex drive. HRT can be taken orally, transdermally through a patch, injected or as a vaginal or transdermal cream. Find a method that best suits your lifestyle as well as your medical needs.

Your HRT is dependent on the type of hysterectomy you had and your risk level of developing breast cancer, heart disease and osteoporosis. If you have your ovaries and if they are actively producing therapeutic levels of estrogen and progesterone, there is a good chance you will not need any HRT. But if you do need it, you and your doctor will have to discuss the right treatment plan. An ideal level should make you feel good and result in healthy bones, cardiovascular health and an overall sense of well-being.

Studies have shown an increase in the risk of developing breast cancer for women using HRT; however, these are preliminary, and more data are needed. As with any health concern, this varies among women.

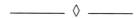

Women who have had a hysterectomy because of endometriosis need to keep a close watch because estrogen can exacerbate microscopic endometrial tissue.

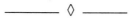

This means that the endometriosis may flourish and return. Progesterone may counterbalance the effects of the estrogen, lessening the risk of recurrence. It is extremely important that you work with a physician experienced in managing HRT and reproductive endocrinology. Estrogen taken alone may increase the incidence of cancer of the endometrium. That's why it is important for some women to counterbalance the effects of estrogen with progesterone.

Hormone replacement therapy can dramatically reduce the ill effects of menopause, such as night sweats, hot flashes, depression, insomnia and vaginal dryness. It is also clear that HRT can help a woman maintain bone mass, which lessens the likelihood of developing osteoporosis, a degenerative disease that effects bone density in post-menopausal women. HRT can also lower a woman's risk of developing heart disease or heart attacks.

Hormone replacement therapy continues to spark debate that can be overwhelming and confusing. Find out for yourself what works. As long as you are not putting your health at risk and working with a physician who is competent and reliable, you can experiment until you find the right HRT for *you*. For the best information, examine your health history and find a physician whom you trust to determine possible benefits and risks.

SIDE EFFECTS OF HRT

We all hear horror stories of women going through hormone replacement therapy and experiencing uncomfortable effects, from mood swings to absence of libido. Usually the side effects of HRT are manageable and become merely a minor annoyance. Estrogen and progesterone have their own set of side effects. Estrogen may elicit nausea, fluid retention, abdominal cramping and swollen breasts, while progesterone can effect moodiness, depression and spotting.

Taking estrogen and progesterone, I felt as if the bottom had fallen out from under my feet. I found myself melancholy and irritable. It seemed like within seconds I metamorphosed from my "normal" state of mind into a raving witch, simultaneously crying and feeling sad. The worst part was that I could not find a trigger for these emotions. What had happened to make me so irritable and sad? I went from enjoying a day of shopping with my fiance to feeling absolutely miserable. Every time I lashed out at him or tried to make sense of what was happening to me, I felt worse. It was a lose-lose situation and it left me feeling confused and upset. (It felt like Lupron revisited!) I immediately consulted my gynecologist as well as a reproductive endocrinologist, and my hormone levels were adjusted. Now we wait and see. Sound familiar?

If I sound bitter, I am not. If I sound weary of being a guinea pig, I am. I am tired of having my hormones "played" with time and again. Although I realize there is no one to blame, it still hurts. I don't ride the emotional roller coaster well. It's bumpy and noisy and unpredictable, and sometimes I want to jump off and leave the park. But the park is life, and we all have to learn to live within its realm.

We are strong women who *can* and *do* forge ahead in search of answers. I know that someday we will find them. Together, hand in hand, we will find them.

~

Chapter Seven

A Man's Perspective: How To Care For Each Other

The repercussions of living with endometriosis extend far beyond the woman who has the disease. It has a tremendous impact on the man in her life. The dynamics of the relationship are radically changed and it can cause major stress on the healthiest of couples. I speak from experience. I know what it is like to feel so much pain and sadness and to have my fiance feel helpless because he desperately *wants* to help but cannot.

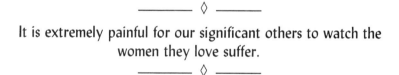

It is extremely painful for our significant others to watch the women they love suffer.

The frustration at not being able to "fix" you is overwhelming, and men tend to either retreat into their own worlds or become overly concerned to the point of suffocation. There is a medium, and I am going to help you find it.

We all know how hard it is to deal with this disease day in and day out. Our physical and psychological selves are constantly challenged. It takes enormous energy to face up to these challenges, and they often leave us physically and emotionally bankrupt. This affords us little or no capacity to participate in our relationships—even with our partner—and can leave a man feeling neglected, angry and frustrated. He wants to know what is happening, why it is happening and how to remedy it. Unfortunately we know that there are no clear-cut explanations for these questions. If we had them, we would certainly share them. But there are ways to ease the burden. First, let's talk about the changes you are both going through.

REOPENING THE LINES OF COMMUNICATION

When we are suffering and in pain, the last thing we want to do is make love, go to the theater or take a walk along the beach with the man we love. We desperately wish we could, but we can't. You need him to understand that the difference between wanting to do something and your ability to do it can sometimes be as day is to night. We need our partner to understand this and not assume he can read our minds or our actions. We need to communicate *with words* the exact nature of our feelings.

Honest, straightforward and continual communication is the key to maintaining a healthy relationship. Expression can be difficult when we are suffering, but we must try. Also, let him express his thoughts, fears and frustrations. He is the other half of the picture—the one so often overlooked or ignored. He needs to know he is not "less than" for not being able to help you, and that you would let him help you in a heartbeat if there were anything he could do. It is the endometriosis—not you and not him.

I know how hard it is to care for the one you love when you can barely care for yourself, but even the smallest of gestures can ease a man's anxiety over your illness.

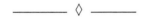

Let him in and let him love you. Let him know how much you appreciate the sincerity of his concerns.

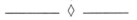

Let him know he is needed, wanted and cared for. Put yourself in his shoes. Wouldn't it make you crazy to watch the man you love suffer, knowing there was nothing you could do to ease his pain?

Here is a letter I received from a man desperately seeking of answers for his wife, who is suffering with endometriosis:

Dear Jennifer,

I am 30 and my wife is 28. We have a son, who is 9. As for any more children, I think we are done. But still the hysterectomy is a hard thing to swallow. My wife was on Lupron for about four months and it did help a little but the side effects were very hard on her.

Her doctor failed to explain all of the bad effects this drug causes.

Do you have the mood swings and depression, hot flashes or any of the other bologna that comes along with the Lupron shot?

It is hard for me to see my wife suffer as she does. It has definitely affected our marriage in ways that are hard to explain: The mood swings from the shot; going from sex three to four times a week to—if I am lucky—maybe once a week or even once every two weeks. Also, our personal life and our party life have stopped. We used to go to our friends' house for barbecues or they would come over to our house. Now it seems that she never wants to do anything, and I guess I don't blame her.

This disease has changed the type of person my wife is. She hurts constantly. I'm afraid to have sex with her even when the chance does come up, and it always hurts. We have been to counseling to get help with this and it has definitely helped.

It's hard to imagine going through life hurting as she does. She takes non-narcotic pain pills that help a little, she says, so this is good that she is not getting hooked on pain-killers. I feel that there has to be more I can do for her.

I try to spend at least an hour a day on the internet e-mailing different doctors or people to help me or her to understand what is going on.

I am not ready to throw in the towel yet.

Thanks.

—Seattle, WA

This man obviously cares a great deal for his wife and feels frustration and fear at being unable to help her. The lines of communication are clearly open, for they work as a team in gathering information and making decisions about treatment and future fertility goals.

HOW ARE WE AFFECTED?

Here is an example:

Dear Jennifer,

Being the husband of a woman with endometriosis is interesting. It is very difficult keeping up with demands I set for myself. I feel like a nurse sometimes. There is a constant reminder that she is sick, let it be her saying so or physical signs of pain. Sometimes I get fed up with it all. I wish I could take it from her but I can't. It's all she talks about and sometimes I just don't want to hear it. I take it out on her when I don't want to hear it and that's wrong.

How can I expect her not to think about it all the time when it is always here?

The bottom line is it's hard to live with even if you don't have it. So how did I get so lucky to find this diseased woman and fall in love with her? Why me? Well it's not her fault and it's not mine. This wonderful woman didn't wake up one day and decide to be sick. It's just fate, I guess, just as our meeting was. Our love will carry us through and I'll be right by her side until a cure or death makes us part.

Caring for somebody is God's work and if she needs somebody to help her through it then I would be honored People shouldn't have to go through pain alone, so be strong! Stand by your woman because she would stand by you.

—Pontiac, MI

Here is a letter from my fiancee, who expresses his feelings and emotions about living with a woman with endometriosis. This is to assure you that I am no different than you are and that we have the same struggles and tribulations.

To my beautiful fiancee, Jenn,

When you asked me to write a letter about how I felt, I was excited and flattered that you wanted my thoughts. I have been wanting to put into words all that I have been thinking and feeling about you and our relationship. I have feelings and although I can never feel the pain as you do, I want to help in any way I can.

I can never express all the love I have in my heart for you. I fell in love with you the day we first spoke and when we finally met I knew I wanted to love you forever. It pains me deeply to sit on the sidelines, wanting to come and rescue you, pick you up on my steed and whisk you away, away from all the pain. I want to make it better, kiss it and make it go away, hold you in my arms and tell you that it will be OK and that soon the pain will go.

As I look reality in the face I realize that I can't make the pain stop no matter how much I want to. What I can do is love and support you and be there for you no matter what happens.

You can be a bitch at times, so mean and hurtful, but is it really me you are angry at? The truth is that the pain and this damn disease have caused you to say and do these things.

Please don't misunderstand me, sweetheart, I love you and I will never stop loving you; it just hurts me deeply. Before I met you I never heard of endometriosis and the hell that it can wreak on a woman's life, as well as her spouse's. I am still learning more each day about this little-known illness and you have helped educate me. I now have an urgent need to learn as much as I can, for you, and for us. What I do know is that it is extremely important to understand what endometriosis is and just how much women suffer. A man needs to give unrelenting support to his partner by doing all the little things that she cannot do because of her limitations, such as cleaning, laundry, cooking, running errands and helping with the kids. He needs to be sensitive tender and understanding and most of all, to love her unconditionally.

I love you, Jennifer, with all that am. My gratitude to God for bringing you into my life is immeasurable. You have fulfilled my life and I love you for the kind, compassionate, loving person you are. Every night I pray that your pain and suffering will subside and allow you the freedom you so much deserve. Just remember, darling, that you are my life and my love and that living without you would be no life at all. We will fight this together, and until you are well, lean on me. I will be there always. Let me be the strength to hold you up when you cannot

All my love,

Michael.

I cried when I read this letter. It's amazing what words can do, especially when they come from the heart.

If you are having difficulty speaking, try writing out your feelings. Even the most stoic of men may surprise you with his words

A woman with endometriosis is not the only person whose life changes. The man who loves her must make psychological, social, economic and physical adjustments. He will have thoughts and feelings about these changes, and it will be essential to remove any communication barriers to fully understand the effect on the relationship.

Depending on the severity, patterns will develop as a result of the disease. If the woman is usually the one who goes grocery shopping or picks up the kids from baseball practice, the husband may take on these responsibilities while she is no longer able to. If she is a primary breadwinner and cannot work, the husband may have to take on another job—or watch the family fall into debt.

There may be hidden resentment from a husband not accustomed to these responsibilities, and guilt from a wife who cannot perform them.

It will take special effort to fully accept the frustrations and limitations placed on both of you.

Your pain affects both of you; try to help each other. Women often feel guilt at not being able to have sexual intercourse. Find alternate ways to express your love. This will enhance your intimacy and expose both of you to alternate, but equally pleasing, solutions. This involves change, and change is sometimes difficult to embrace. The ability to adapt to change and to acknowledge what you can and can't change will reduce the feelings of inadequacy and helplessness.

He is human, and his reactions to your illness may vary. Don't be alarmed if he balks at first when you discuss how much you bleed or that it hurts like mad when you try to have a bowel movement. He may be unaccustomed to talking so frankly and openly about your gynecological health. If this is happening, remind him that endometriosis *is* a hard disease to explain without these explicit terms and that you don't like having to deal with this disease, either. Also, give him credit. He may not embrace this topic with the passion that you have; his capacity for dealing with this may not match yours. Give him time to adjust to the changes in your situation, and help him to understand your feelings about the adjustments.

Unfortunately, there are men who are less than helpful or downright negligent and refuse to take on additional responsibilities. This can make you feel unloved and hurt and can cause major rifts in your relationship.

———— ◊ ————

Take it slow, give him a little time without compromising your health or self-esteem.

———— ◊ ————

If you think he does not have compassion for your pain, think again. He may be angry and frustrated at not being able to help. At the root his of anger is fear. He fears losing control, losing the life he is accustomed to and, most of all, losing you. He fears change. Change can be threatening and uncomfortable. Anticipate changes in

Remember, he is not angry with you, but the endometriosis.

If your partner refuses to communicate, let him be and focus on *you*. Find a support group or a friend who will listen.

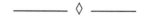

We do not always get the support we deserve from those people we assume will be there for us.

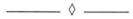

Although this is disheartening, we still need to forge ahead and seek the help we need.

TOOLS FOR COPING

Learning how to manage your feelings and behavior takes work and practice, especially as a couple. Work together to understand what works and what doesn't in your communicative styles. Many times we greatly affect others' emotions and responses without even realizing it. Here are examples of commonly used words or phrases and other alternates:

Instead Of Saying	Practice Saying
"You shouldn't do that"	*"I prefer you not do that"*
"You never help me"	*"You rarely help me"*
"You have to understand"	*"I want you to understand"*
"You are always moody and irrational"	*"I can see you are upset, what can I do to help?"*

Instead Of Thinking	Try Thinking
"I must"	*"I prefer"*
"I should"	*"It is desirable"*
"I can't stand"	*"I don't like"*
"You always"	*"Oftentimes"*
"ought"	*"had better"*
"have to"	*"choose to"*

This small change in your use of vocabulary can dramatically alter your communication by removing blame and reprisal. Using "I feel" statements instead of blame and reprisal. Using "I feel" statements instead of "You are" statements can help make both of you feel more comfortable. Little changes can make a huge difference.

A LETTER TO THE MAN I LOVE

Often, we are so consumed with our illness that we forget to reassure our loved one that we do indeed love, want and need him. Here is a sample letter to the men we love and who love us:

To the Man I Love,

I write this letter because oftentimes my actions (or lack thereof) contradict the way I feel about you. This is not intentional. My love and respect for you gets overshadowed by my constant pain and struggle with this horrible disease. I see how much you hurt when I am hurting, and I know you are frustrated at not being able to "fix" me. I understand more than you know. As much as I retract into my own little world when I am suffering, know that your mere presence is always very comforting, nurturing and desired.

Yes, there are many times when I do not wish to be touched but it is not because of you, it is because when I hurt as much as I do I cannot do anything else but focus on my pain. I would love nothing more than to be able to fall into your strong arms and let you make love to me, but I can't. Know that I need you and want you and that you are still my knight in shining armor. You save me with your tenderness, your understanding and your empathy, the aspects that make you far stronger than anyone else in my eyes.

I will always need your love and your intimacy, even if we have to redefine what that is for the time being. Your understanding makes me love you more and more each day you are there with words of comfort or gestures of love. You take care of me and stick right by my side through painful surgeries and horrible medications, through mood swings and crying fits. Through thick and thin, you have never left my side. For that, I am eternally grateful, and for that, I love you more than words can say.

Thank you.

Perhaps this will help you communicate with your loved one, after all, successful communication goes both ways.

~

~Chapter Eight~

Personal Stories of Strength, Courage & Hope

In compiling research for this book, I spoke with, wrote to and corresponded with several thousand women, each with her own story. I was touched by their desire to share some of their most intimate experiences and soon realized that I was not the only one they were confiding in—they were communicating with every woman who has endometriosis. Their cumulative stories provide a base to which other women in need of strength and knowledge can turn to and realize they are not alone. These women offer the greatest gifts of all—their truths, journeys, pain and suffering. And, they provide opinions, options and first-hand experience involving every aspect of dealing with endometriosis, from symptoms and diagnosis to complete hysterectomy.

This portion of the book is dedicated to those who still suffer, who can relate to even one experience provided here, and who will find the courage to seek help. In the interest of privacy, the entries are anonymous.

~

Dear Jennifer,

I want to thank you for your time and effort in gathering information. I am just starting my journey on how to live and deal with endometriosis. I'm still trying to decide if it was better not knowing what was wrong with my body. Please keep up the good work, we need you.

~ London, England

~

~

Dear Jennifer

I am having my first laparoscopy this Tuesday. I will be 22 next month and I am scared to death that I won't have children. The doctors say that is a possibility. I would love to hear back from you. I know so little about this and am scared to death right now.

~ Los Alamitos, CA

~

~

Dear Jennifer,

I have endometriosis and I have had it for years. I am 36 and have always had painful menstruation. Last Friday, I finally had a laparoscopy to prove that I have severe endometriosis. The last four years have been especially miserable, getting worse each year. I have gotten to the point where I am not much good to my own family let alone trying to do things outside my home. I had wanted the doctor to be able to do a hysterectomy as soon as he saw the endo because I know of its rate of recurrence when it is severe. My husband's insurance won't allow such a thing. I am so frustrated with the whole thing. The doctor told my husband that he believed it could have been prevented from becoming so severe if they had done a laparoscopy years ago. That's about it, I guess. I am starting to feel somewhat better after the laser treatment but am skeptical because they couldn't take care of it all.

~ Flagstaff, AZ

~

~

Dear Jennifer,

Hello, I am a 19-year-old and I was just diagnosed with endometriosis. My case started about three years ago. At first I was having abdominal pain on my right side. My doctor thought that I may have had cancer; it runs in my family. I had tests done and they were all negative. Then, last year, the pain moved to my lower abdominal area. My doctor thought I had ovarian cysts but the test for that came up negative as well. Then in May of 1996 I began to get very ill. I got nauseous every time I ate, was constantly in pain and my bowels were not functioning properly. I went from weighing 110 pounds to 92 pounds. My doctor got another gastrointestinal test done this December but like all the others tests it came back negative. I had been to a gynecologist, but he found nothing in any of my pap smears. Finally, I stood up for myself and got a new OB-GYN. He checked everything out and upon physical examination found some scar tissue on my insides. He diagnosed me with endometriosis. Now I am scared because children are my life. If I can't have my own I don't know what I am going to do. What if I can't have them? I am so very scared. Thank you so much for listening.

~ Boulder, CO

~

~

Dear Jennifer,

I saw your message up on the Endometriosis Support Board and thought I would take you up on your offer of support. I would love to talk with someone who is my age and going through the same stuff as I. In the last four months I was diagnosed with ovarian cysts, severe endometriosis and had surgery six weeks ago. My doctor then told me after the surgery that mine was the worst case of endometriosis she had ever seen and three weeks ago I began Lupron shots. She says my chances of having children are basically non-existent.

I have dealt with chronic, horrible pelvic pain for about seven years and painful periods since I was a teenager, but to have this information thrown at me recently is so overwhelming. I am so discouraged because it sounds like I will be back to Square One when I go off the Lupron and just be in for more pain, more problems and an eventual hysterectomy. I feel like my whole body is totally screwed up and I feel unhealthy and depressed about never having children of my own. Is there any chance that this Lupron will help me or am I just biding time?

I am also very depressed because I am not working right now and these medical bills are piling up and Lupron is very expensive. My doctor is good and I like her, but she doesn't seem to have time to discuss these things in depth with me so I am hoping to find answers from others. Thank you for bearing with me and reading this. I appreciate very much any information or advice you can offer.

~ Anoka, MN

~

~

Dear Jennifer,

Hi! Yesterday I just found out that there is a good possibility that I have endometriosis and I am scared out of my mind. I've done all the reading about it, but it has not helped me feel any better. How did they find out that you had the disease? You must have been pretty young. I am 20 years old and am not ready to handle something like this. I'd appreciate if you could tell me how you were diagnosed and dealt with this at a young age.

~ Boston, MA

~

~

Dear Jennifer,

Good morning! Wow, that is awesome that you have written a book about this mystery disease. I call it that because I can never get a clear idea of what exactly endometriosis is. I do not know whether I have it. I have symptoms of something, but no one can put their finger on it. When did you first notice symptoms? Were you always tired during your cycle? I feel as though all the iron and vitamins and nutrients have been sucked out of me. I must rest. I can barely put one foot in front of the other.

I have read about lower abdominal pain and backache. This I have as well, though not to disabling levels like other women. Lately, I have several blood clots during my cycle and evidence of "tissue." I have been told as well that this is par for the female course. Does any of this sound familiar to you? I applaud your courage to take the time to write the book. Thank you for your strong ray of hope to other women who are mostly silently suffering.

~ Paris, France

~

~

Dear Jennifer,

As you know, where does one even begin to talk about the hell we go through. There are so many things that happen to us that only we understand. I am a student and I am 28. I have been trying to get through school for a long time. I was overtaken by pain in April 1996 and then diagnosed in May. I had my laparoscopy during finals and had to take incompletes in two classes and fail another. The hard part is that I have no insurance and I am 100 percent dependent on financial aid. My graduation has had to be pushed back as the fall of 1996 semester has been painful as well.

I am being treated with Lupron and have gone through four shots. I just announced to the doctor today that I cannot stand the side effects anymore. I have dropped two classes and have taken an incomplete in one. I can barely afford the fee per injection anyway. My family cannot help due to illness and no insurance of their own. I hope to graduate in August 1997, but am worried that I will be unable to meet all my financial obligations with an entry-level position. I do not even have a car and do not know how I will get around. Public transportation is time consuming and, as we know, this is a draining disease.

Like so many others, my affliction has affected my relationship with my boyfriend. Sex has no joy for me now. I have no desire for it at all, and it only ends in cramps or pain. I already suffer from clinical depression and endo and Lupron don't help!

I have had, while being treated with Luporn, digestive problems, headaches, hair loss, weight gain, vision problems, exhaustion, skin problems, memory loss, sleep problems, elimination problems and God knows what else is inside of me. I used to be in touch with my body. Now I feel it is just an alien body I have been dumped in. I do not feel attractive anymore and fear that I may not be able to rid myself of the fat that has deposited itself on my hips, thighs, buttocks and tummy.

Who am I? What is my body saying to me now? Is this my body? Why? Why? Why? I have been surfing the Net and wondering if I may have endometriosis in my intestines. One woman's account sounded similar to some symptoms I have suffered. Did my doctors look close enough? Why did my doctor not remove the lesion I have on the right uterosacral ligament.

I have learned more through the internet than through my own doctor.

I learned that there are stages of endometriosis (from I-V). Why didn't my doctor mention this to me? When I asked one of the nurses she said there was no such thing. Are there no standards? Is everyone running around throwing their ideas in the air for whomever to catch?

I have so many questions to throw at my doctor when I see him again. So much is on my mind, I feel I may be on overload. I look for strength in God, my family and women such as yourself. Thank you, Jennifer, and good luck with everything.

~ Las Vegas, NV

~

~

Dear Jennifer,

I have had endo for at least the past two years. I had an ovary and a tube removed due to a cyst the size of a peach in my right ovary. My left ovary is also damaged and my doctor said that the only way to cure my pain is to have a total hysterectomy. I am so tired of feeling terrible for a week to 10 days out of every month. Lately, I have been suffering from terrible nausea the first two days of my period.

I would love to hear if anyone else has or is also feeling this way from endo. I went to three doctors who diagnosed me with PID, uterine cancer and mental problems before I found a wonderful doctor who, upon examination, said I probably had endometriosis. This was even before the laparoscopy! She was right! My advice to everyone is don't be afraid to get a second opinion. Find someone that you trust!

~ Boca Raton, FL

~

~

Dear Jennifer,

I am so sorry you have had such a bad time of things at such a young age. When people tell me they feel bad for me for having had a partial hysterectomy I realize there are others out there who may be experiencing the same problems without having the chance to realize all of their dreams.

My problems began after I had my tubes tied with a banding process in 1992. I had just had my second child and I knew that I was happy with my family and didn't want to have any more children. The doctors that I used to do the tubal ligation were the same doctors that delivered my second child so I had faith in them and their abilities and medical experience.

As it turned out, four days prior to my surgery I got my period and thought they would have to reschedule my surgery. I called my doctor's office and they told me that having my period would, in no way, affect my surgery and that we could continue as planned. The day of the surgery, I again asked my doctor if it was O.K. to tie my tubes while I was having my period. He said that it was O.K. Having been reassured, we proceeded with the surgery.

Two months after the surgery I started having pain on my lower right side. The pain seemed to be related to my period and got worse and worse month after month. There were many calls to the doctor's office looking for answers and help. Finally in May of 1995 I had my first exploratory laparoscopy and the doctor, a new one, could not find much, but he cauterized and cut the right tube. This is when the possibility of endometriosis was discussed. I had some adhesions and he addressed those but the pain continued.

I was on every kind of pain medicine out there, but in the end, even demoral couldn't dent the severe pain.

I finally found a new doctor who specialized in endometriosis.

This was the first time a hysterectomy was suggested. I balked at the suggestion and when at home, convinced myself that this doctor was "cut happy." But then I got my next and last period. It was brutal and I called my doctor crying and scheduled the surgery.

Two days after the surgery I got the pathology reports that were positive for adenomyosis, endometriosis in the uterine muscle. The recovery from the laparoscopy-assisted vaginal hysterectomy was slow and painful.

What was even more painful was finding out on my own that my endometriosis was definitely triggered by the first doctor tying my tubes while I had my period.

The endometriosis cells migrate and behave much like cancer cells and some cells migrated during my tubal surgery, implanting themselves in an area that they should not have been in, causing pain.

Before I had my tubes tied, I was a normal, healthy, fertile woman who had two full-term babies, with normal periods and no history of any problems. I am now a 36 year-old woman who feels different from all my friends and at times, depressed. I thought you should hear my story.

I believe that my endometriosis did not have to happen, and now I have a cyst on my right ovary and recurring endometriosis. The doctors are watching me very carefully. Thank you for allowing me to share my story. It is terrible feeling like a victim, but by telling you my story, if it helps another woman make different choices, then it will make me feel better.

~ Syracuse, NY

~

~

Dear Jennifer

I have been lurking around the Endometriosis Support Board for about a month. I have one daughter (23) who has been diagnosed with endometriosis, Stage III-IV, and another (28) who is due for a diagnostic laparoscopy soon. I laughingly refer to myself as a "mother lode of info on endo." Neither of them have access to the Internet so I have been reading, and reading, and reading. Your posts have been very helpful for someone like me.

As a mother, the hardest thing imaginable is to see your children in pain and be unable to "fix" it.

I haven't seen too many posts from the people who love the women with endometriosis. As much as I try, I can never feel their pain or suffering. I wish you all the success with your book.

~ Cambridge, Canada

~

~

Dear Jennifer,

I have suffered from endometriosis for more than ten years. I have had more than twenty surgeries and have been treated with every medicine imaginable, including those for irritable bowel syndrome; I have been on Lupron six times!! Instead of getting better, I keep getting worse.

At this point, I barely leave my house any more for fear of having an "attack" of pain. Work has suffered, my marriage has suffered and my life as a whole is suffering. The pain is debilitating and constant and I am in search of support and information as to what else can be done to make it *go away*. Good luck with your book.

~ Baltimore, MD

~

~

Dear Jennifer,

I'm in the same boat you are! I have had endometriosis since I was 15, but I was "diagnosed" during spring break of last year. So now I am starting to turn this "thing" that happened to me into a good thing!

I am starting an endometriosis support group at the school I am attending.

Talking about school, all last year my grades dropped significantly. I transferred here in the spring and was totally excited to be in a four-year, rather than two-year, college. But I was in so much pain I had to drop out of dance, missed other classes or couldn't concentrate because of the pain. My spring break was spent "recovering" from the three-hour laparoscopy. Finals were the following month and to make matters worse, the Percocet did nothing to ease the pain, it only made me dizzy. I ended up with a C in history, a D in chemistry and the following semester I failed my genetics class, dropped out of physics and got a C in statistics. I begged my professors to give me incompletes, but they were unsupportive.

The problem was that I was letting the endo be a handicap and letting "it" beat me. I have changed my major to an easier one so I won't be so overwhelmed. The Web has been a lifesaver; I can get all sorts of information on this subject!

~ Bowling Green, KY

~

~

Dear Jennifer,

Your letter brought tears to my eyes. When I looked up your profile I kept thinking, why am I feeling so terrified and so sad at the loss of children that I possibly could not have anyway due to my age? Your courage and candor are greatly appreciated. I have been putting this off for so long, waiting to meet Mr. Right or Mr. You'll Do. When I lived with my last boyfriend for five years we didn't use birth control for over six months; I think I figured that if I got pregnant then I would deal with it. I was 37 then and that biological clock was overwhelmingly loud. Now, at 42, when it's just about wound down, I should be able to handle this with a bit more maturity.

I'm just so scared about the hormones, my sexuality and my "femaleness." I can't explain it but I am sure you understand. Did you have a weird sort of panic start to sink in prior to your hysterectomy? It's two months away but I keep thinking that I only have two periods left…this is so dumb…all they have ever meant to me is severe pain and nausea, and yet I am grieving over losing them.

I'm not in a relationship right now and I am not sure if that is good or bad. The whole thing just scares me. Do you feel the same as you did before? Did you take hormones or the patch? Did you feel as lost as I do right now? I keep thinking that this could be cancer or some other truly-life threatening disease and that I should just "get over it" and stop whimpering.

I'm only whimpering internally; I try to preserve the I've-got-it-together and have worked-it-out front. Now if just one more friend could stop saying, "Don't do this yet" or "Maybe they will come up with something in the next couple of years."

Anyway, sorry for the long-winded response, the subject makes me pretty emotional and I really appreciate your shoulder. I've had pain since my first period due to endometriosis, but the pill took care of a lot of it. I am so sorry that you had to go through this when you did and I truly admire your courage and sensitivity. Thank you.

~ San Francisco, CA

~

~

Dear Jennifer,

I am 33-years-old and have had endometriosis for many years. I, too, have had two unilateral oopherectomies that left me in surgical menopause, and five laparoscopies in the last four years. I have been on Lupron, birth control pills and many others. I *had*—and I repeat *had*— a gynecologist who promised after each surgery I would have no problems ever again. When they found endometriosis on my ureter and iliac structure and the Lupron didn't work, they actually suggested Prozac.

I have a new doctor who is kind and caring, but I still think I know more about this than he does.

My wish is to find a doctor who I don't have to educate.

I was put through too many surgeries and they feel it's too risky to go back in. I suffer more from adhesions though and because of Lupron I can add joint pain to my many symptoms. I have had it. I want answers, too.

~ New Orleans, LA

~

~

Dear Jennifer,

I'm really frustrated! I had surgery for endometriosis for the first time a year and a half ago. My doctor said it was the worst case of endometriosis he had ever seen. I really don't remember a time when I was completely without some kind of pain when it came time for my period. I'm now in constant pain. It's been going on for about three months but I wouldn't go to the doctor because I knew I was going to have to go through everything all over again. It took six months for the doctors to decide I had endo in the first place.

They did every test imaginable and I repeatedly got looked at like there was nothing wrong with me.

It was like they didn't believe I was in pain because they didn't see anything.

I remember being so frustrated and crying all the time because I was beginning to really feel like I was going crazy.

I had laser surgery followed by six months of Lupron shots.(I hate needles!) I was also diagnosed with Irritable Bowel Syndrome but that miraculously went away after the surgery and the shots. I finally went to my family doctor yesterday and she diagnosed me with Irritable Bowel Syndrome (again) and said that she thinks the endo is "back." That's how it all began the first time.

She wants me to go to the Ob-Gyn who did the surgery and have him check it out. I really don't feel like I am strong enough to do this. I can't imagine having to go through this every year and a half. I'm trying to talk to friends and family around me and it is just like they don't understand how upset I am. I really want to just lay down and cry but I know that's not going to make it go away.

It really makes me feel not so bad to find other people who have some kind of the same problems that I have.

I'm married and want only my two children so they can just give me a hysterectomy so I can be rid of this whole thing. But you still have pain after hysterectomy, so how does one know what she is supposed to do? Thanks for sharing your story with everyone. You have a great web page!

~ Dayton, OH

~

~

Dear Jennifer,

Thank you for the time you spent writing a book about endometriosis. I have had endo since I was 13 and just had surgery at 30. I still have complications and look forward to reading your book. It's nice to know there are people out there who care enough to share their wealth of knowledge on something doctors can't cure.

~ Long Island, NY

~

~

Dear Jennifer,

My daughter just turned 15 in January. She is going in for a laparoscopy this Friday. It may be endometriosis. It sounds like you were diagnosed at age 17. What have your independent, real-world respondents had to say about the age factor? I keep hearing that 15 is awfully young to have developed endometriosis.

I'm so afraid for Friday to come. If the Lap is positive for endometriosis then I'll cry, knowing what is ahead for my little girl. If it is negative, then I'll continue to be frustrated until we can figure out where this almost constant pain is coming from. The pain is in her lower left abdomen.

The ultrasound done three weeks ago was negative. She started her period in the fifth grade (young) and so heavy was the bleeding, one "period" lasted for ten weeks. She is now in the ninth grade and has been on the pill for about six months, which slowed the bleeding a lot but the pain has increased dramatically.

She is active, in cheerleading and drama, gets good grades and has lots of friends. She is handling this better than I am. My mom, sister and I have had hysterectomies for various reasons; mine due to adenomyosis. I am so hopeful that we can get some answers on Friday. Wish us luck!

~ Miami, FL

~

~

Dear Jennifer,

Yesterday I was diagnosed with endometriosis. I am not sure what it really means. I am doing research but am just getting dry facts. I want to know how it affects the women who live with it. My mother had it, but they did a hysterectomy on her in 1986 and discovered it was endometriosis, afterward.

I have been getting the horrible cramps with my period since it started when I was twelve years old. I have had my colon and rectum removed for a chronic degenerative disorder called Crohn's disease. I now have an ileostomy.

Anyway, my pediatrician tried me on the basic over-the-counter pain medicines, then I switched to a family doctor when I was 14 and he gave me the same stuff only a little stronger. (During all this I had a couple more abdominal surgeries due to Crohn's.)

The one I have been taking for the last year has been Vicodan, which does nothing but make me able to move enough to get to school, except for the first two days of my period when I can barely leave my bed without crying from pain or getting nauseated. My mother suggested I see a gynecologist, which at 15, scared me to death. I saw her and she said that I had endometriosis. She also said that because of my ileostomy and other surgeries she could not do a laparoscopy because it is too dangerous.

She is starting me on the pill for a few months to see if that helps. I have been reading about some of the other medicines they use to treat this and the meds scare me. I haven't found anything yet to say whether having endometriosis means I will never have kids. I am just frightened that my options will be closed when I am only 15. Oh well, thanks for listening.

~ Saratoga, CA

~

~

Dear Jennifer,

I am so sorry you had to have a hysterectomy at the age of 27. I had a hysterectomy at 41 after twenty years of the same symptoms and complaints to doctors. I did not know I had endometriosis all those years. From the age of 15 I had lower right quadrant pain all the time and at 19 I was told I had an ovarian cyst. I started having two periods a month.

After the birth of my first child I asked the doctor why I always hurt and he said, "tender ovaries," and if it got really bad they could be removed. Of course, I said no. I was only 23 and wanted another child. Needless to say this went on for years.

I had the second child and continued the same symptoms of pain, two periods, diarrhea and all the rest. I really don't blame the doctors. As a nurse I know it wasn't understood that well. When I was sent for a pelvic sonogram the results were positive and the surgeon diagnosed endometriosis and I wound up with a total hysterectomy and oopherectomy.

I have loved the last fourteen years of no pain and I feel great! Good luck with your book, there are many women out there with this problem.

~ Little Rock, AK

~

~

Dear Jennifer,

I have recurrent endometriosis, have had four surgeries already and am having my fifth this week (pain mapping where you are semi-awake). Unfortunately it is in the doctor's office so equipment will not be available to take care of a problem right then, so surgery number six is on the horizon.

Yes, it hurts like hell sometimes, but I don't give up! I had to go through five doctors in my area and finally went to my sixth, sixty miles away. This is the second time he is going in for me.

You just have to keep going and find that one doctor who will continue to believe you.

Only *we* know what we feel and that the pain is the same as before. We know that we are right even though you may doubt yourself when they say it's all in your head. Don't stop following your instinct. You don't have to put up with the pain forever, someone will believe you. We all hope for a cure. Best of luck on search for yours!

~ Santa Barbara, CA

~

~

Dear Jennifer,

I have had endometriosis since I was 16 and I am now almost 24. I have already had five surgeries, been on Depo-Provera among other hormonal drugs and pain pills. A year ago I had surgery and the doctor was going to cut a nerve and I was supposed to be pain free for five years, well last month I started having pain *again!*

I want to have children someday, but right now my husband isn't ready to be a daddy. I want children so badly I am afraid that I won't be able to have them when he is ready. I am running out of things to try.

I just started looking this up on the internet tonight and now I don't feel so alone. Thank you.

~ Shreveport, LA

~

~

Dear Jennifer,

I have endometriosis. I just found out about two years ago and it took them two years to finally diagnose me. I went through ten doctors.

I have been on Lupron and I had a baby and now it's back again. The doctor wants to put me on more medication. I don't know what to do at this point. I don't know who to talk to or where to get support so I am hoping you can help me.

I am 25. I asked my doctor to give me a hysterectomy and she said it would not help me because my endometriosis has spread. I feel at a loss here. I was then told I would be on hormones for fifty years if I had a hysterectomy, but it seems like I will be on pain meds and drugs for the rest of my life without one. Can you help me?

~ Detroit, MI

~

~

Dear Jennifer

I am sorry to hear about your recent hospitalization due to endometriosis. Don't tell me that it doesn't mimic cancer cells.

I believe that endo behaves just like cancer and if they started treating it as if it were as deadly as cancer, then there would not be a stigma attached to it.

It may not *kill* us, but it maims us and destroys our bodies, our lives and our family's lives also.

I still have pain on my lower right side and until it is killing me I won't even call the doctor. I am even tired of people asking how I feel. I just don't want to be the "sad sack" anymore.

~ Atlantic City, New Jersey

~

~

Dear Jennifer,

I had a full hysterectomy in 1994 due to severe endometriosis. I was sick with cramps since I was 12 or 13. My family knew how much I suffered but none of the doctors they took me to diagnosed the problem as endometriosis. They gave it other names, other medicines and sent me home.

So little has been written and is truly known about it. I have cried myself to sleep many nights.

We need to demand more research and a different method of training for our gynecologists.

Most have thought me to be mentally unstable, hysterical, acting out or just overemotional. I am hoping that there is a miracle out there that will help me live the remainder of my life normally and without pain. Maybe you have found it.

~ Oxford, CT

~

~

Dear Jennifer,

I am 16 and have endometriosis. I have had five surgeries within the last year and have tried birth control, Depo-Provera and Lupron twice. I have gone to many different doctors and don't know what to do next. I would have a hysterectomy, but I am too young and I want to have kids. Do you have any suggestions?

~ Kona, HI

~

~

Dear Jennifer,

I am 27 and battling endometriosis. I have become very frustrated in my treatment. Thankfully I have two beautiful children but the disease is destroying my life. I have had surgery twice in the past four months, been on birth control pills, taken Lupron and am now battling the choice of taking yet another hormone, Danazol. I had surgery three weeks ago and am back to square one in extreme pain.

I find that living my life constantly taking narcotics and over-the-counter medications to be getting very old, but that is the only way I can seem to cope with the pain. All of the treatments thus far have gotten me nowhere but more depressed and frustrated.

I went to my doctor today with my husband to discuss where we go from here and it seems the only option left is to have a complete hysterectomy. I am very torn with this as I dreamed of having another child. My husband is trying to be supportive but has great difficulty understanding how we have done all these treatments and I am still in so much pain, not to mention the other symptoms.

I feel so alone in all of this.

I have a wonderful family but no one can understand what I am really going through. I feel as though I am backed into a corner. It is all so unfair; life is not always fair. I know this, but this is almost more than I can bear.

How do I get past these emotions? I finally feel that I have found someone who will not consider me crazy or that this is all in my head. I would appreciate anything you can tell me and anywhere you can lead me to learn more about this disease that has consumed my life. Thank you so much for your web site and your concern for others.

~ Richmond, VA

~

~

Dear Jennifer,

I was searching the internet today and came across your page. After surgery in December I was told that I have endometriosis. So far, I have been taking the birth control pill and now, Lupron. I'm 23 and have had problems since I was 13. Nobody really understands.

Before I had the surgery my doctor basically told me I was a mental case or had been sexually abused.

He could not understand why I was having painful sex— and those were his answers since he could find nothing. I wish I could talk to someone who understands this disease. I am excited about your book.

~ Lununberg, Nova Scotia

~

~

Dear Jennifer,

I am 23 and was diagnosed with endometriosis in November 1996. The world is really so much more difficult since endo took over my life. I never had a difficult period. I never had any cramps until right before I was diagnosed. Then one day out of the blue I became really sick. Within five minutes the cramps in stomach were so severe I could not breathe in or out. My left leg shot pain from my pelvic area to my toes. I could not stand or even crawl to the phone to get help.

Finally, when I did get to my doctor, who, by the way, I credit all my information to and couldn't imagine life without, I had the laparoscopy. I started Lupron in December which was eight days after my surgery. They started it to slow down my bleeding. Then came the mood swings and the weight loss and the emotional outbursts, the list goes on and on.

Currently I am going for my fourth Lupron shot next week. I take 20 mg of Prozac a day, have .05 Climera estrogen patch and if I have a great day, only two to four 100mg. of Darvocet or Tylenol with codeine a day. (Prozac for the mood swings, Climera for the cramps and pain killers for those oh-so-pleasant headaches.)

How do I feel about Lupron? I hate it with all my heart!! But, my body reacts to birth control pills the same way and I am not stable enough to bring a child into this world, so there is no other option. I am a strong believer that things happen for a reason, and if God intends for me not to bear a child—so be it. There are too many children out there with no families who need love and attention. I'll just scoop up one of them and go on about life!

I will note one thing about women with endometriosis; though we go through so much pain and suffering that is so unbearable at times, we remain strong.

Yes, we cry when the cramps and pain come, and yes we get emotional, depressed and aggravated, but we are still out there trying to understand why and teach others about this condition. It's hard, God, I know, but we're all in a boat and we all have to paddle just as hard to get to the cure of this thing.

So, Jennifer, I wish you and your book a wonderful success. Stay focused on the good things in life and remember, no matter what, even if you try, you can never be alone in this world. Take care and best wishes.

~ Orlando, FL

~

~

Dear Jennifer,

I live in Australia and for some time now I have been experiencing very severe period pain and pains in my bowel when I am menstruating. I also lose a great deal of blood, more than I ever have before. I am unable to walk, clean or talk normally when the pain is happening. I am getting really sick of it.

Are these symptoms of endometriosis? I will have to have exploratory surgery to find out and then treatment I guess. Do you know if these symptoms are indicative of anything else? I would really like to hear form you!

~ Sydney, Australia

~

~

Dear Jennifer,

I also have the dreaded "E". I had an ovarian cyst removed in January of this year and am currently taking Lupron…and I'm still in pain all the time!! It seems like my doctor doesn't even believe me,

She gives me Bentyl and smiles and says it'll go away, yeah right! I'm thinking of finding another gynecologist but I'm not sure, at least she figured out what I had wrong! The three doctors I went to before her did not find anything.

Oh excuse my crankiness; I had a very bad night. Please e-mail me and let me get to know someone who understands. I don't know how much longer I can take this. How have you managed for ten years? I can't even imagine.

~ Oakland, CA

~

~

Dear Jennifer,

I just got done reading your page on the web. It's nice to know I am not the only woman in the world dealing with this problem. I've known that I've had endometriosis for over three years now. The doctor said that I could have had it as a teenager. I always had problems with my periods but never thought anything of it. I thought it was what was natural. Who would have known it would take over my life as it has?

It has hurt me with my jobs, losing so much work time due to pain. It has put a damper on my relationship with my family members, friends and my boyfriend.

I thank God I have a strong boyfriend who understands, but it still isn't easy. He can't stand seeing me in pain.

I've had three surgeries, the last was exploratory only. I'm on my fifth going on my sixth month on Lupron. This is my second time on this treatment. The first was only for three months. I've also been on Synarel for a short time three years ago. I am not experiencing much pain right now, but I am also not working right now.

Every time I get stressed-out, the pain comes flooding back. I've been told by three different doctors that I need to have kids before it's too late and have a hysterectomy after I am done having children. My boyfriend and I plan on getting married in about a year and are thinking of trying for a baby early. My doctor wants to put me on Serophene fertility pills so I get pregnant faster.

I don't know what to do anymore. Every time it comes back it comes back harder and stronger. I'd appreciate any answers you could give me. I heard that it is not good to go on hormone replacement therapy for three to nine months after having a hysterectomy. I'm sure you have heard this already but I thought you should be aware just in case.

~ Pontiac, MI

~

Dear Jennifer,

I have endometriosis and I hate it! I was diagnosed last year after years of pain and infertility. At first I was relieved to know what the problem was, but now I am so frustrated by this disease. I ended up in the emergency room in January and now I am on Lupron injections.

Lupron is a nightmare! I don't know which is worse, the endo or the Lupron. I'm having a lot of hot flashes and headaches, and the mood swings—they've been awful. I've finally found someone who understands how devastating this disease is.

~ Toledo, OH

~

~

Dear Jennifer,

I am 23 years old and I was diagnosed with endo when I was 21. It's only been a couple of years but it sure has been a long haul. I have had surgery twice, changed the dosage on my birth control pills, changed doctors, seen specialists and nothing has changed.

My present doctor would like me either to get pregnant or try Lupron for six months before attempting any more surgery. Although I'm engaged, getting pregnant is not an option. I'm young and I would really like to have time to enjoy life, although in my present condition I'm not really having that much fun.

I'm skeptical of Lupron. I'm looking for information on the effects of Lupron while taking the shots. Of course, my doctor has given me pamphlets but I'm looking for information from women that have had to face the same decisions that I am.

I want to know what could really happen to me if I go through with the Lupron course. Will I be any better after the six months? Will I feel the same way that I do now and regret having gone through the Lupron therapy?

I enjoyed your home page. It is really comforting to know that there are other women around the world that I can talk with about this problem. It's nice to know that I'm not alone.

~ St. Paul, MN

~

~

Dear Jennifer,

I wanted to thank you for your web pages. I am at the end of my rope and have tied the knot. I am trying to hang on, but things seem to be getting worse. My doctor's appointment is on the 19th of May. I have been on birth control pills but my prescription ran out three weeks before my appointment, so I am not taking anything and the pain is just getting worse by the minute. Do you have any tips for ignoring the pain?

I have had problems with adhesions and from all the research I have done I am almost positive I have endometriosis. Thanks for being there and allowing me to vent. I hope all is well for you. Take care and thanks again.

~ San Diego, CA

~

~

Dear Jennifer,

I had a total hysterectomy and oopherectomy seven years ago and felt great at first. I now think that was because it took a while for all the natural hormones to leave my body. Then I was hit with severe mood swings, from anxiety to depression and back again. I had never before had any mood swings so this was frightening.

I have tried many hormonal treatments and I can't say that any is perfect but I have come to kind of an uneasy truce with it all and manage to live my life with enjoyment most of the time. It is really a drag though to have the mood problems that come from surgical menopause. Not everyone seems to get them and I have a theory that it may be people who are especially susceptible to changes in their neurochemistry. I have always been very affected by any drug and I think that it worked both ways in the sense that when my own hormones were taken out of my body I also reacted more strongly than many do.

Unfortunately I had no idea that this would be a problem and was quite cavalier about having my ovaries removed. I often wish I could make that decision again. However, I have tried most things that are recommended and actually find that best of all is careful diet (no sugar, little fat and many small meals throughout the day to keep blood sugar even), adequate sleep, regular exercise and meditation. When I do these things every day my mood stays more even.

I also did well for awhile on Estratest but had to quit because it made my cholesterol high. The patch gave me a headache and Premarin seems okay, but the side effects build up and I have to go off every once in a while. I like using the natural progesterone cream to kind of clean out my system for the estrogen, so every once in while I go off estrogen and do that for a week. Sometimes I'd like to go off it all but I seem to sort of crash when I do that.

I still try new things because I am always looking for better HRT that more approximates my old feeling. The first year or two were harder because the body does do some adjusting. I still don't like the way it is now but it is a lot better than it was initially, so that's the good news!

~ Santa Monica, CA

~

~

Dear Jennifer,

I am 21 and had my hysterectomy nine months ago. I got endo at 12 and it took several years to diagnose because of my (young) age. I went round and round to many doctors until I finally found someone who helped me. I had pain twenty-four hours a day, seven days a week for nine years.

I am now out of pain; prayerfully that will continue. There is no guarantee that I will stay this way but I hope women who are new to this disease don't give up too quickly. I want women to understand that there still is hope. I hope your book helps others like us. Thank you for being there and good luck.

~ Long Beach, CA

~

~

Dear Jennifer,

I am finally scheduled for another laparoscopy. This is after one Lap not even a year ago and a hysterectomy less than six months ago.

The doctors said that it was impossible for the endometriosis to return after a hysterectomy.

I had to go through so many wild goose chases and drugs without results to get to this point, it's been like pulling eye teeth to get them to take another look! I know it has returned, wish me luck!

~ Santa Fe, NM

~

~

Dear Jennifer,

They did the surgery and guess what they found? Endometriosis!

~ Santa Fe, NM

~

Dear Jennifer

I will be having a hysterectomy this week. I have had endometriosis for six years and my last laparoscopic surgery two years ago. The laser surgery barely lasted six months, my condition progressed to adenomyosis. I have three kids and am 31. I am anxiously looking forward to recovering and coming back stronger than ever!

~ Jacksonville, FL

~

~

Dear Jennifer,

I, too, have had several laparoscopies and a total hysterectomy for severe endometriosis. Currently, I am completely off hormones and I am still having severe pain during intercourse only. I've been battling this for six years and I am completely frustrated.

My doctor thinks the pain is in my head and is thinking about referring me to a psychiatrist.

How is it that pain so severe cannot be treated completely?

~ Houston, TX

~

Dear Jennifer,

I will probably have the hysterectomy at the end of this month and I am actually looking forward to getting it over with and getting on. I have been consumed with this for quite a while and it will be great to get past this and focus on better health. I have been married for seven years and each year we renew our wedding vows. This past year we vowed, "In health...for richer...." We feel that we have had enough of the "In sickness...for poorer...." I typed it up in big letters and it hangs on our refrigerator. I am looking forward to that! I feel confident in my decision. Thanks!

~ Des Moines, IO

~

~

Dear Jennifer,

I am 26 and have had endo since I was 17.

I have had nine surgeries, two neurectomies, two nerve blocks, removal of my right ovary and appendix and countless other procedures. Surgery number ten is scheduled for this summer.

I have tried all the usual meds (Lupron, birth control pills, etc.), as well as herbs and other natural products. I am in a pain management program and they have shown me how to give myself Demerol and Vistril injections when I get my period.

I think that I have just about exhausted all of my options besides a hysterectomy. I would really appreciate any advice that you could share with me. Thanks for reading this. Take care.

~ Boston, MA

~

~

Dear Jennifer,

I guess I really need to talk to someone who has endometriosis. I'm upset because today I told my GP that I went to the ER early this morning for pain, and he said, "Now your menstrual pain should not send you to the ER." This upset me greatly because I thought he was the one doctor who understood my pain.

He went on to say that he has never known anyone who has had to go to the ER for menstrual cramps, and that endo shouldn't cause me so much pain that I can't control it.

Could you please send me e-mail to tell me whether you have had to go to the ER for your endometriosis pain? I would love to be able to print it and then show it to my doctors.

Thank you in advance,

~ Charleston, NC

~

~

Dear Jennifer,

I am 27 and recently I was told that I have endometriosis. I decided to look on the web for help and that is when I found you. I am really thankful that I found your page and hopefully some one I can quiz about what is going on with me.

Since I was 16 I have had severe abdominal pain. The doctors chalked it up to cramps and I was given countless pain medications. I believed all of it until last year on my honeymoon. I miscarried, and I did not even know that I was pregnant. A few months later the cramps got worse and intercourse hurt. Finally, last week I decided to put aside my embarrassment and ask questions of my newest gynecologist. She examined me and for the first time, I heard the word endometriosis.

I am nervous about my upcoming laparoscopy, but am excited to get this behind me and move on. I realize I do not know you, but I really felt a connection with your page and wanted to tell you how much I appreciate your comments.

~ Wichita, KS

~

~

Dear Jennifer,

I found out that I had endometriosis when I was 18 and having my gallbladder removed. I thought that I would feel much better after the surgery, but finding out I had endo made me so upset. I was never told the full details of this disease and I thought I would never be able to get pregnant. I never had any of the signs so it seemed impossible that I could have it. But then the pain started and I became very moody. Is there no hope of ever getting over this? I'm scared of not being able to get pregnant when the time comes. Do I need to be worried? My doctor gave me some medication for the pain but it does not help. What kind of medication really works? For me, having endometriosis is really scary simply because I never heard of it before my diagnosis and was not told all the information.

Will I ever not be scared of this stuff that is growing inside of me? I am scared and unsure.

~ Memphis, TN

~

~

Dear Jennifer,

I came across your home page today and am very interested in talking to you. I am 32 and have had endo for five years.

It took many doctors two years to finally diagnose it, telling me I had everything from arthritis of the sternum to stress or that it was my imagination.

I have had three surgeries and just finished my sixth and final injection of Lupron. The pain is starting to come back.

Did you ever find a pain killer that actually stopped the pain? My doctor is reluctant to give me more than a stronger form of Tylenol which does nothing when the pain is severe. I'd love to hear more of what you have found. I feel helpless sometimes and my husband feels the pain is all in my head.

~ Northridge, CA

~

~

Dear Jennifer,

I am 21 and found out this past Wednesday that I have endometriosis.

I am still in shock but so relieved that I finally have a name to go with the pain.

Right now I am just trying to get all the information about endo. My main concern is kids. I have always wanted lots of kids, and now it seems my dream is gone.

I did not know that so many women were afflicted with endometriosis. It amazes me how I never heard of this until Wednesday. I had pain since I was 14 and always had irregular menstrual cycles.

I feel relieved and also scared. If you have any information that you would be willing to share I would appreciate it. Thank you for your time, your page is wonderful!

~ Dallas, TX

~

~

Dear Jennifer,

I feel like I am losing my mind. I am crying as I type this.

I am 32, married and am in almost constant pain. The pain is focused on my lower right side and lower back. It is not just mild pain, it is debilitating at times. I can't do ordinary tasks when this happens, even bending over can be a killer. I had an ultrasound and other minor tests and only "residual inflammation" was found. I have been to four different doctors in five years and none of them have seemed too concerned or interested in my plight. None of them have suggested a laparoscopy, they have only unofficially diagnosed me with endometriosis.

How long have I had this pain? It sure seems like forever. It has been ten years at least and is getting progressively worse. My family says it is "in my head." I guess because there has been no actual diagnosis (laparoscopy). No one in my family has endometriosis. Does it have to be hereditary? My husband and I have tried to conceive for seven years. No luck.

I tried to work out the other day when my side and lower back just "locked up" on me. I thought I would die right there and then. I just laid on the bed and cried.

No one understands how this affects my life. My husband is a gentle, wonderful man but how can he begin to understand the frustration and pain that is becoming such a vast part of my life? I am really beginning to believe I am going crazy. Do the doctors truly even care?

~ Billings, MN

~

Can you identify with any of these women? Do you have more questions than answers and feel that you need to be more of a participant in your health care? Are you satisfied with the treatment you are receiving?

You may be angry with the health care you are receiving and have unmet expectations. Turn that anger into assertiveness and your expectations into reality. Let your doctors know what you expect from your relationship. Do they know already? If not, write down ten expectations of your optimal doctor-patient relationship. After that, share them with your physician.

He or she may not be aware that you are so frustrated, and I have learned that being angry will not help the situation. Be assertive and make your expectations clear as well as a reality.

~

~Chapter Nine~

Your Diary

This portion of the book is for you—to help you begin keeping a health log. Only after ten years of living with endometriosis did I finally become aware of the importance of keeping my own records. Yes, doctors have your records on file, but since they treat hundreds of patients, their records are not anywhere near as accurate as they could be.

Also, if you move or change providers, your own records will be a lifesaver to both you and your new doctor, enabling treatment to readily begin. We all know the perils of having our records transferred! Why take the risk? It is your responsibility to help yourself by keeping accurate records of your own. This is part of the job of being an advocate for your own overall health.

Included are samples of my own Medication Journal, Treatment Timeline Journal and Symptom Journal. Also provided are forms to help you begin your own journals. Please make copies or create your own forms. Keeping a log of your medications, your responses to them and your questions about them will help prepare you for your next doctor's visit or alert you to a problem, such as nausea with a specific medication, and that you should call your doctor about immediately.

JENNIFER'S MEDICATION JOURNAL

Medication/ Dosage	Physician	Date	Why Started
1 Elevil 50mg	Dr. Red	5/1/96	Sleep deprivation
2 Premarin .625	Dr. Yellow	8/29/96	HRT/ Hysterectomy
3 Vicodan 500 mg	Dr. Green	9/4/96	Post-Op pain
4 Prozac 20 mg.	Dr. Blue	12/8/96	Mood swings

Comments & Side Effects— Are These Medications Working For Me?

1. The Premarin is to help with side effects of surgical menopause. But I am still having hot flashes and night sweats. I also have vaginal dryness. Be sure to bring this up with Dr. Yellow at next appointment.

2. I am having trouble staying asleep at night. I can fall asleep O.K. but I always wake up in the middle of the night and cannot get back to sleep. The Elevil is to help me sleep, perhaps I should call Dr. Red.

3. I have read that one of the side effects of Prozac can be agitation. I have been feeling anxious and jittery. Talk to Dr. Blue.

A record of your treatment and your feelings about it is helpful to you and your health-care team. This is discussed in Chapter Four. I have kept a record like this one since 1991.

YOUR MEDICATION JOURNAL

List All Your Prescription Medications Here

Medication/ Dosage	Physician	Date	Why Started
1)			
2)			
3)			
4)			
5)			
6)			

COMMENTS AND SIDE EFFECTS
Are These Medications Working For You?

1)

2)

3)

4)

5)

6)

JENNIFER'S TREATMENT TIMELINE JOURNAL

Date	Treatment	Comments
4/22/96	Pap Smear	Call for results
4/28/96	Pap Smear	Abnormal. Scheduled for Colposcopy.
5/6/96	Colposcopy	Abnormal pap. Feel sore. Call Tues. for results.
5/17/96	Office visit	I am scared. Dr. says tests were positive for cervical dysplasia stage two. Don't really know what this means.
6/27/96	Office visit	Severe pain and excessive bleeding. Dr. ordered blood tests and examined me. Dr. seemed to be annoyed by my questions and pain.
7/7/96	Office visit	Blood test normal. I'm having trouble urinating. I have not been able to go for more than fourteen hours. Nurse catheterizes me and wants me to learn to do it myself. I say no because I am in such pain. Dr. angry that and won't self-cath. I want to know why I can't go.

Documenting your pain and symptoms is crucial in obtaining an accurate diagnosis and receiving effective treatment. In my journal, I wrote down where and when my pain and/or symptoms occur. I try to be as specific as possible.

YOUR TREATMENT TIMELINE JOURNAL

Keep a journal of your treatments as discussed in Chapter Four

Date   Treatment   Comments

JENNIFER'S SYMPTOM JOURNAL

Date	Symptoms
4/1/96	Having severe pain in lower-right quadrant. Hurts all the time.
4/7/96	Heavy period. Went through ten Tampax in one day. Abnormal amount of blood.
4/15/96	Still bleeding and cramping is severe, especially in lower right quadrant. Vicodan is ineffective in relieving the pain. Heating pad helps a little. Nausea.
4/24/96	Spotting with sharp, shooting pains up vagina and down right leg. Painful intercourse.
4/24/96	Bleeding after intercourse. Pain.

YOUR SYMPTOM JOURNAL

Be as Specific as Possible When Listing Your Symptoms

Date   Symptoms

~

~CHAPTER TEN~

HELPFUL RESOURCES

For better or for worse, we are all in this boat together, and we must help one another stay afloat. There are stormy seas and heavy winds, and we may slip and fall overboard, but we are each others' life preservers. We must help everyone climb back in and forge ahead.

There is a future for us. A future of no pain and no suffering. A future filled with happiness and joy. A future with a cure.

This chapter is to inform you about resources on endometriosis. These include organizations, support networks and support groups, hotlines, newsletters and books. Some resources are accessible through the internet. Electronic and postal addresses are listed where appropriate.

———— ◊ ————

You are not alone. Reach out and explore the many resources listed and find some that suit your individual needs.

———— ◊ ————

They are here to help you find out more about endometriosis as well as provide support and comfort.

ORGANIZATIONS

American Association of Gynecologic Laparoscopists
1301 E. Florence Avenue
Santa Fe Springs, California 90670
Phone 1-800-554-2245
Fax (562) 946-0073
E-mail: generalmail@aagl.com

American Association of Obstetrics and Gynecologists
2915 Vine Street, Suite 300
Dallas, TX 75204-1069
Phone: (214) 871-1619
Fax: (214) 871-1943

American College of Obstetricians and Gynecologists
    (ACOG)
409 12th Street, Suite 10
Washington, DC 20024-2188
Phone: (202) 638-5572

Atlanta Reproductive Health Centre
285 Boulevard NE., Suite 320
Atlanta, GA 30312
Phone: (404) 265-3662
Internet site: http://www.ivf.com

Endometriosis Care Center
4575 North Shallowford Road
Atlanta, GA 30338
Internet site:
    http://www.mindspring.com/~perloe/ecc.html

Endometriosis Research Center & Women's Hospital
751 Park of Commerce Drive, Suite 130
Boca Raton, FL 33487
Phone: (561) 988-0767
Fax: (561) 995-7121
E-mail: EndoFL@aol.com

Endometriosis Treatment Program
St. Charles Medical Center
2500 NE Neff Road
Bend, OR 97701
Phone: 1-800-446-2177

National Health Information Center
Phone: 1-800-336-4797

Endometriosis Association
8585 North 76th Place
Milwaukee, WI 53223
Phone: (414) 355-2200
Fax: (414) 355-6065

The National Endometriosis Society
Suite 50, Westminster Palace Gardens
1-7 Artillery Row
London SW10 1RL, U.K.
Phone: (44)-171-222-2776
Fax: (44)-171-222-2786

BOOKS, PERIODICALS & NEWSLETTERS

Mary Lou Ballweg. *Endometriosis Sourcebook: The Definitive Guide to Current Treatment Options, the Latest Research, Common Myths About the Disease.* Lincolnwood, IL: Contemporary Books, 1995.

Winnifred B Cutler. *Hysterectomy: Before and After: A Comprehensive Guide to Preventing Preparing for and Maximizing Health After Hysterectomy.* New York: Harper Collins, 1990.

Amy Gross and Dee Ito. *Women Talk About Gynecologic Surgery: From Diagnosis to Recovery.* New York: HarperPerennial, 1992.

Susan Lark. *Fibroid Tumors and Endometriosis Self Help Book.* Berkeley, CA: Celestial Arts, 1995.

C. O.Truss, M.D. *The Missing Diagnosis.* n.p.: Missing
Diagnosis, 1985.

Kate Weinstien. *Living with Endometriosis: How to Cope
With the Physical and Emotional Challenges.* New
York: Addison-Wesley, 1995.

Endometriosis Research Center Newsletter
Phone: (561) 988-0767
Fax: (561) 995-7121
$10.00 annual fee/ newsletter published monthly

St. Charles Endometriosis Newsletter
Phone: 1-800-486-6368
Free/ quarterly

Endometriosis Association
Phone: (414) 355-2200
$35.00 annual fee/ monthly (irreg.)

Vital Signs
UCLA Medical Center
Free/ monthly

ONLINE RESOURCES

Jenn's Endometriosis Homepage!
http://users.aol.com/bucalu/index.html

Endometriosis Resources
http:// www.goecites/Hot Springs/1712/endo.html

Endometriosis Frequently Asked Questions
http://www.stayhealthy.com/hrd/dicopr_reurco_
enis.html

Atlanta Reproductive Health Centre
http://www.ivf.com

Endometriosis Information and Links
   http://www.frii.com/~geomanda/endo/

Endometriosis Care Center
   http://www.dunwoodymed.com/endo/endocare.
   html

~

~APPENDIX~

PHOTO SECTION

   While each woman's diagnosis is unique, much about endometriosis is shared by those who have experienced it first-hand. The following seven photos depict the most common areas of the body where endometrial implants occur.

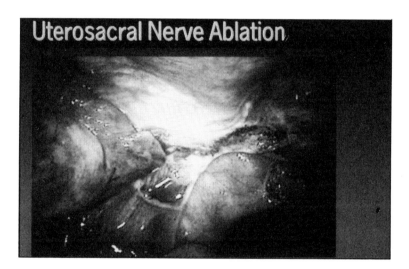

Uterosacral Nerve Ablation

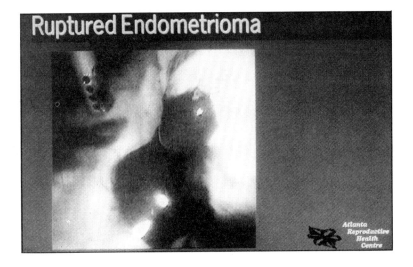

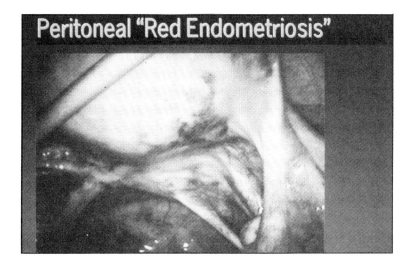

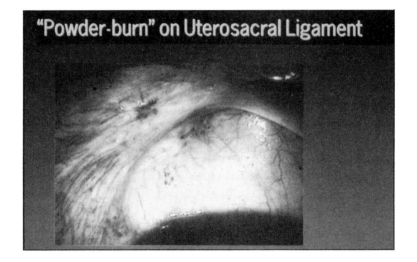

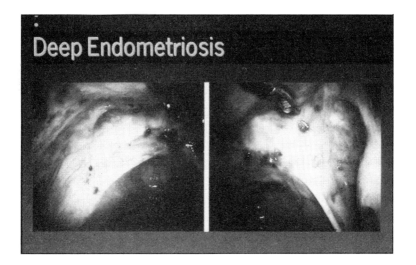

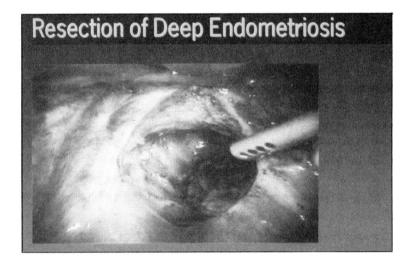

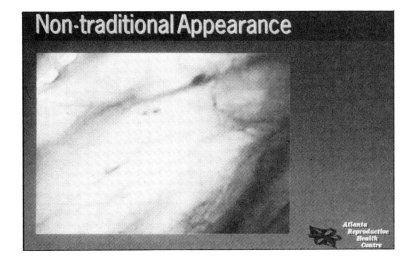

~

A Word From The Author

What a journey it has been, and it is far from over. Through our shared experiences we have discovered a new ray of hope—ourselves. You might be a mother of three, a student, a doctor, nurse, teenager, homemaker, lawyer, or schoolteacher. One thing we have learned is that endometriosis does not discriminate. Hence, it is imperative that all women unite in becoming their own health advocates. This is your body, your sacred self. Place your physiological or psychological health only in the best of hands—yours and those of a professional who has earned your trust and respect.

Endometriosis is our commonality and our past. It now becomes our journey into the future. What kind of journey it will be and where it will take us no one knows. I do not know where to find keys to unlock this and so many other doors of unanswered questions. Until I have the answers, I will diligently continue searching—for all of us.

~

~

Jennifer Lewis is available for individual personal support related to endometriosis. Fees are negotiable. Jennifer writes a column for the Endometriosis Research Center Newsletter (See the "Helpful Resources" section for more information).

The author may be reached through her publisher at:

Griffin Publishing Group
544 Colorado Street
Glendale, California 91204

Telephone: (818) 244-1470
Fax: (818) 244-7408
e-mail: griffinbooks@earthlink.net

Jennifer's website:
    http://users.aol.com/bucalu/index.html

Griffin Publishing's website:
    http://www.griffinpublishing.com

~INDEX~